The LONGEVITY SOLUTION

Rediscovering Centuries-Old Secrets to a Healthy, Long Life

DR. JAMES DINICOLANTONIO
& *Wall Street Journal* Bestselling Author **DR. JASON FUNG**

Victory Belt Publishing
Las Vegas

First Published in 2019 by Victory Belt Publishing Inc.

ISBN-13: 978-1-628603-79-8

Author photos by Megan DiNicolantonio and Dean Macdonell

Cover design by Justin-Aaron Velasco

Interior design by Elita San Juan and Charisse Reyes

Printed in Canada

TC 0119

CONTENTS

PREFACE

A Note from Dr. DiNicolantonio

In my previous two books, *The Salt Fix* and *Superfuel*, I tackled several long-standing nutritional fallacies, particularly the forty-year-old lies that salt is bad for you and vegetable oils are good for you. *The Longevity Solution* builds upon these works by exploring the mysteries of mTOR, dietary protein, and calorie restriction and looking at the dietary habits of the healthiest humans on the planet to unlock the secrets of healthy aging. *The Longevity Solution* also covers the benefits of intermittent fasting, collagen and glycine, green tea, coffee, and red wine. Finally, Dr. Fung and I lay out five easy-to-follow steps for a longer, healthier life.

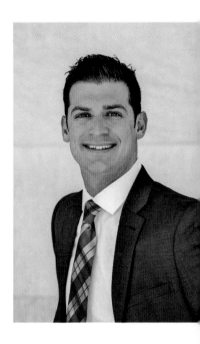

Perhaps you believe that following the government's Dietary Guidelines for Americans, with its familiar mantra of less salt, more vegetable oils, and more carbohydrates, will keep you healthy. Unfortunately, my years of cardiovascular research and Dr. Fung's years of practical clinical experience have convinced us that this dietary advice is almost completely wrong. For example, eating meals based on highly refined carbohydrates will put you in a perpetual cycle of high and low blood glucose that keeps you hooked on these foods (a state known as carbohydrate dependence). The Dietary Guidelines also neglect to mention that the Japanese and other long-lived Asians tend to eat high-salt seafood dishes and avoid refined vegetable oils—doing the exact opposite of the U.S. government's recommendations.

Simple dietary changes can help you break the cycle of carbohydrate dependence, kick your metabolism into high gear, and jump-start your longevity genes. Intermittent fasting is a great example of one such simple change. Fasting resets your metabolism, allowing new, better cells and proteins to replace older ones. This "out with the old cells, in with the new" process of self-repair is called autophagy, and increasing autophagy through fasting is just one "biohack" that might help extend your life span as the body is busy with self-repair instead of growth, which promotes aging. Other dietary patterns commonly found in long-lived populations, such as drinking red wine, tea, and coffee, are easy to follow and improve both health and longevity.

Let *The Longevity Solution* be your official guide to improving your health with simple, easy changes to your diet and lifestyle that you can start implementing now! Activate your longevity genes and start promoting cellular repair rather than cellular despair.

A Note from Dr. Fung

People often believe that the secrets to longevity lie in the newest gee-whiz technology or the latest, greatest supplement. Paradoxically, the secrets to healthy aging have been communicated to us for centuries, and sometimes millennia, as they've been handed down from generation to generation. *The Longevity Solution* rediscovers these ancient lost secrets—and shows how they're supported by what we now know about biology. Recent research has uncovered the science behind ancient longevity-promoting practices such as restricting calories; optimizing dietary protein; drinking tea, coffee, and red wine; and eating more salt and natural fats. The more things change, the more things stay the same.

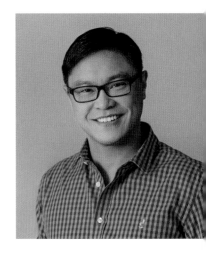

These ideas are not the latest and greatest fads. They are tried and true. They have been used since antiquity and were traditionally accepted as important facets of wellness. Ancient peoples knew that they worked, but modern science is just now figuring out the reasons behind their success. These secrets have been hiding in plain sight. We just didn't know where to look.

People are always searching for what they can add to their diet to extend life and improve health. Over the years, the list has become endless. Supplements of vitamins A, B, C, D, and E have been touted as the next great cure-alls. One after the other has failed, sometimes miserably. The problem is that we're not asking the right questions. In addition to asking "What do I need to eat more of to get better?" we need to ask "What do I need to eat less of to get better?" *The Longevity Solution* asks both questions—and, more importantly, answers them.

01

AGING:
NATURE DOESN'T CARE HOW LONG WE LIVE

The legendary Spanish conquistador Juan Ponce de León (1460–1521), like many of his bloodthirsty contemporaries, sought fame and fortune through exploration of the New World. He settled in the part of Hispaniola that is now the Dominican Republic, before serving as the governor of Puerto Rico for two years. When Christopher Columbus's son, Diego, replaced de León, he was forced to set sail once again. He had heard native tales of a fountain that would restore youth to anyone who drank from it. As part of his next phase of exploration, Ponce de Léon searched for this elusive source of longevity.

He explored much of the Bahamas and is believed to have landed near the present-day town of St. Augustine in northeast Florida in 1513. He named this "newly discovered" land Florida, from the Spanish word *florido,* meaning "full of flowers." He continued his explorations throughout the Florida coast and the Florida Keys but died never having found the elusive fountain of youth.

This well-known story is likely entirely fictional. Ponce de León's writings make no mention of his search for the fountain of youth, and his vigorous explorations were for more pedestrian reasons—to find gold, identify lands for colonization, and spread Christianity. But the notion of a mystical substance that can reverse aging is so powerful that this legend has endured all these years. Interestingly, the legend of a fountain of youth predates de León; similar stories are part of the Middle Eastern, medieval European, and ancient Grecian cultures. Can aging really be reversed? Has science succeeded where Ponce de León failed?

What Is Aging?

Let's start by looking at what aging is. Everyone instinctively knows what it means to age, but to successfully tackle any problem, science requires an accurate definition. We can view aging in several ways.

First, aging is often obvious because of a change in appearance. Gray hair, wrinkled skin, and other superficial changes signal age. These physical changes reflect underlying physiological changes, like decreased pigment production in hair follicles and decreased skin elasticity. Cosmetic surgery changes appearance but not the underlying physiology.

Second, we can view aging as a loss of function. Over time, women have decreasing fertility until ovulation eventually ceases completely during menopause, in a process largely determined by age. Bones become weaker, increasing the risk of breaks such as hip fractures, which are problems we rarely see in young people. Muscles also become weaker, which explains why champion athletes are invariably young.

Third, at the cellular and molecular levels, response to hormones decreases with age. For example, high insulin (a fat- and glucose-storing hormone) or thyroid hormone levels won't benefit you much if your cells no longer respond to those hormones. Mitochondria, the important cellular components that produce energy and are commonly known as the "powerhouse of the cell," become less efficient and less able to produce energy. The declining efficiency of an aging body results in higher rates of illness and disease.

Increasing age exponentially increases the risk for disease and death. Heart attacks, for example, are virtually absent in children but common in the elderly. Aging is not a disease itself, but it increases the chances of developing diseases, which makes it the best target to stop or reverse chronic diseases. Age, in chronological years, is a river—irreversible and flowing in a single direction. But *aging*, in physiological years, is not. Many factors contribute to aging and disease, and in this book, we primarily consider the aspects that are influenced by diet.

Given the overall functional decline, why do organisms age at all? In short, aging is the accumulation of damage. Young animals, including humans, have a high capacity for repairing the damage of everyday life, such as when children scrape their knees. Species' survival depends on the ability to repair this damage: for example, in healing wounds or broken bones. With age, this ability to repair damage diminishes in all respects—whether it is to fight infections, clear arteries, or kill cancer cells. But this decline is not a natural, foregone conclusion. Nutrition and lifestyle determine much of the speed and extent of the aging process. Long-lived, healthy populations around the world that eat few processed foods show us the possibility of slowing the aging process.

Hippocrates, the ancient Greek father of modern medicine, long ago acknowledged nutrition as the cornerstone of health and longevity. Famine is one of the Four Horsemen of the Apocalypse, but the modern problems of obesity, insulin resistance, and diabetes are equally deadly. In both cases, the foods we eat play an important part in promoting or preventing all these issues.

One important damage-repair mechanism is called *autophagy*. (The fact that the 2016 Nobel Prize in Medicine was awarded to Yoshinori Ohsumi for his "discoveries of mechanisms for autophagy" underscores how vital this process is.) In autophagy, cellular parts called *organelles* are broken down and recycled periodically as part of a wide-ranging quality control system. Just as a car needs regular replacement of oil, filters, and belts, a cell must replace its organelles regularly to maintain normal function. As cellular organelles pass their expiration dates, the body ensures that old organelles are removed and replaced with new ones so that no residual damage impedes function. One of the key discoveries of the last quarter century is that the foods we eat heavily influence these damage control procedures.

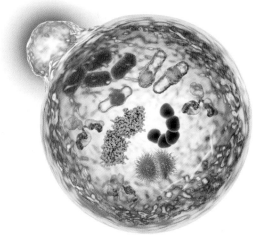

Evolution Doesn't Care Whether You Age

You might think that evolution would perfect our damage control responses, allowing us to live forever. But evolution doesn't care if you age or even if you survive. It ensures the survival of the *species*, not the *individual*. Once you've had children, your genes will survive even if you don't, so there is no natural selection toward longer-lived species. This reasoning is behind the theory of aging known as *antagonistic pleiotropy*. Despite its name, the theory is relatively simple.

Evolution by natural selection works at the level of genes rather than for individual organisms. We all carry thousands of different genes and pass them to our children. Genes best suited to the individual's environment survive better and enable the individual to produce more offspring. Over time, these beneficial genes become more widespread in the population. Age plays a large role in determining the effect of a gene on the population.

A gene that is fatal at age 10 (before a person has children) is rapidly eliminated from the population because the person bearing that gene is unable to pass it on. A gene that is fatal at age 30 will still be eliminated (albeit more slowly) because people without that gene have more children. A gene that is fatal at age 70 might never be eliminated because the gene will have passed into the next generation long before it manifests its deadly effects.

Antagonistic pleiotropy suggests that genes have different effects at different stages of life. For example, a gene that increases growth and fertility but also increases the risk of cancer in old age means more children but a shorter life span. This gene would still spread in a given population because evolution favors survival of the gene, not the longevity of an individual life. One gene might have two different, unrelated effects (pleiotropy) that are seemingly at odds with one another (antagonistic). Survival of the gene is always given priority over longevity of the individual.

This particular gene described codes for a protein known as insulin-like growth factor 1 (IGF-1). High levels of IGF-1 promote growth, allowing organisms to grow larger, reproduce faster, and weather wounds better. That's a huge advantage in the competition to survive in order to have children. However, in old age, high IGF-1 contributes to cancer, heart disease, and early death, and by that time, the gene has already passed into the next generation. When growth/reproduction comes up against longevity, evolution favors reproduction and high IGF-1 levels. This is the fundamental and natural balance between growth and longevity.

Viewed in this manner, the fight against the ravages of aging is a fight against nature itself. Aging is completely natural, although the extent and speed are variable. Living and eating completely in tune with nature does not prevent aging. Nature and evolution do not "care" about your longevity; your genes' survival is the only concern. In a sense, we must look beyond nature to slow or prevent aging.

Aging and Disease

Shockingly, and almost without precedent in human history, children today might have shorter life spans than their parents.[1] The twentieth century witnessed huge and steady advances in medicine and public health that significantly increased average life expectancy. But recently, an epidemic of chronic diseases is threatening to reverse that enviable record.

Before the modern industrial era, with its advances in sanitation and medicine, infectious diseases were the main natural causes of death. In the United States in 1900, life expectancy at birth was 46 years for a man and 48 years for a woman, due largely to high infant and childhood mortality.[2] But those who survived childhood had a good chance of surviving to older age. The top three causes of death in 1900 were all infectious diseases: pneumonia, tuberculosis, and gastrointestinal infections.[3] These infectious diseases can affect people at any age, although children and the elderly are especially vulnerable.

Today's situation is different. The top two causes of death are cardiovascular disease and cancer, and both diseases correlate tightly to age. Cardiovascular disease, which includes heart disease and stroke, is the number-one cause of death in the United States, accounting for one in four deaths, and its incidence increases dramatically with age.[4] Children rarely suffer heart attacks, but by age 65, the majority of us have developed some form of cardiovascular disease.

The story is the same for cancer. Children and young adults each account for only about 1 percent of new cancer cases each year.[5] Adults aged 25 to 49 account for about another 10 percent, whereas people aged 50 and older account for around 89 percent of all new cancer cases. Other diseases with clear links to aging include cataracts, osteoporosis, type 2 diabetes, Alzheimer's, and Parkinson's. These diseases of aging are responsible for approximately two-thirds of the roughly 150,000 deaths that occur around the world every single day. These are diseases that affect hardly anyone younger than the age of 40. In the industrialized West, the proportion of people who die from aging-caused diseases approaches 90 percent.[6]

As modern medicine conquered infectious diseases like smallpox, one consequence of this success is an aging population with its inherently higher risk of chronic diseases. But that's not the whole story. The seemingly unstoppable and unparalleled obesity epidemic is putting our health at increasing risk of cancer and heart disease. There are many dietary and lifestyle modifications that you can adopt to reverse this risk of chronic disease.

Aging is the slow accumulation of cellular damage due to a decreasing ability to repair it. The result is a low level of inflammation, which is so characteristic of aging that it's been termed *inflammaging*. Oxidative stress, a condition in which free radicals (highly reactive molecules with an unpaired electron) overpower the body's internal antioxidant system, rises with age. However, you can make lifestyle changes that can increase your odds of healthy aging. You can increase not just your life span, but your "health span." Nobody wants to spend their last years frail, sick, and in a nursing home. The prevention of aging is about more years of healthy life during which you're free of disease and other drawbacks of old age, you feel vigorous and energetic, and you have an enthusiasm for living. Longevity means extending youth, not extending old age.

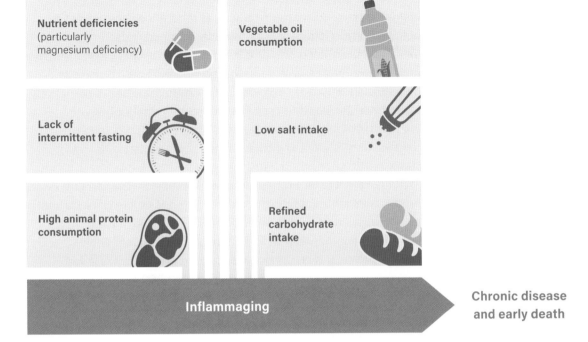

Nutrient deficiencies (particularly magnesium deficiency)

Vegetable oil consumption

Lack of intermittent fasting

Low salt intake

High animal protein consumption

Refined carbohydrate intake

Inflammaging

Chronic disease and early death

Fig. 1.1: Causes of inflammaging

Evolutionarily Conserved Mechanisms

Simple one-celled organisms called *prokaryotes*, such as bacteria, are the earliest forms of life on earth and are still abundant today. *Eukaryotes*, more complex but still single-celled organisms, first appeared approximately 1.5 billion years later. From those humble beginnings came the multicellular life forms called *metazoans*. All animal cells, including in humans, are eukaryotic cells. Since they share a common origin, they bear a resemblance to one another. Many molecular mechanisms (genes, enzymes, and so on) and biochemical pathways are conserved throughout evolution toward more complex organisms.

Humans share approximately 98.8 percent of their genes with chimpanzees. This 1.2 percent genetic difference is enough to account for the differences between the two species. It might be even more surprising to learn that organisms as far apart as yeast and humans have many genes in common. At least 20 percent of genes in humans that play a role in causing disease have counterparts in yeast.[7] When scientists spliced more than 400 different human genes into the yeast *Saccharomyces cerevisiae*, they found that a full 47 percent functionally replaced the yeast's genes.[8]

With more complex organisms, such as the mouse, we find even greater similarities. Of more than 4,000 genes studied, fewer than ten were found to be different between humans and mice. Of all protein-coding genes—excluding the so-called "junk" DNA—the genes of mice and humans are 85 percent identical. Mice and humans are highly similar at the genetic level.[9]

Many aging-related genes are conserved throughout species, enabling scientists to study yeast and mice to learn important lessons about human biology. Many of the studies cited in this book involve organisms as diverse as yeast, rats, and rhesus monkeys, and they vary in the degree of their similarity to humans. Not every result applies to humans, but in most cases, the results are close enough that you can learn a great deal about aging from them. Although it is ideal to have human studies, in many cases these do not exist, which forces us to rely on animal studies.

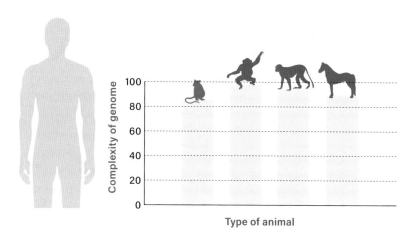

Fig. 1.2: Genomic similarities between humans and animals

Theories of Aging

The following sections outline the principles of several theories of aging and our verdict on the plausibility of each.

DISPOSABLE SOMA THEORY

The disposable soma theory of aging, originally proposed by University of Newcastle professor Thomas Kirkwood, holds that organisms have a finite amount of energy that can be used either in maintenance and repair of the body (soma) or in reproduction.[10] Like antagonistic pleiotropy, there is a trade-off: If you allocate energy to maintenance and repair, then you have fewer resources available for reproduction. Because evolution directs more energy toward reproduction, which helps propagate its genes to the next generation, the individual's soma after reproduction is largely disposable. Why devote precious resources to living longer, which doesn't help to pass on the genes? In some cases, the best strategy is for the individual to have as many offspring as possible and then die.

The Pacific salmon is one such example; it reproduces once in its lifetime and then dies. The salmon expends all of its resources for reproduction, after which it tends "simply to fall apart."[11] If there's little chance that a salmon would survive predators and other hazards to complete another round of reproduction, then evolution will not have shaped it to age more slowly. Mice reproduce quite prodigiously, reaching sexual maturity by two months of age. Subject to heavy predation, mice allocate more energy to reproduction than to fighting the deterioration of their bodies.

On the other hand, a longer life span may allow for the development of better repair mechanisms. A 2-year-old mouse is elderly, whereas a 2-year-old elephant is just starting its life. In elephants, more energy is devoted to growth, and they produce far fewer offspring. The gestation period of an elephant is eighteen to twenty-two months, and the result is only one living offspring. Mice produce up to fourteen young in a litter and can have five to ten litters per year.

Although it's a useful framework, there are problems with the disposable soma theory. This theory would predict that deliberate calorie restriction, which limits overall resources, would result in less reproduction or a shorter life span. But calorie-restricted animals, even to the point of near starvation, do not die younger— *they live much longer*. This effect is seen consistently in many different types of animals. In effect, depriving animals of food causes them to allocate *more* resources to fighting aging.

Further, the females of most species live longer than the males. Disposable soma would predict the opposite because females are forced to devote much more energy to reproduction and thus would have less energy or resources to allocate to maintenance.

> **Verdict:** It fits some of the facts but has some definite problems. The disposable soma theory is either incomplete or incorrect.

FREE RADICAL THEORY

Biological processes generate free radicals, which are molecules that can damage surrounding tissues. Cells neutralize them with antioxidants, but this process is imperfect, so damage accumulates over time, causing the effects of aging. Large-scale clinical research trials show that supplementation with antioxidant vitamins like vitamin C and vitamin E may paradoxically *increase* death rates or result in worse health. Some factors known to improve health or increase life span, such as calorie restriction and exercise, increase the production of free radicals, which act as signals to cells to upgrade their cellular defenses and energy-generating mitochondria. Antioxidants can abolish the health-promoting effects of exercise.[12]

> **Verdict:** Unfortunately, some facts contradict the free radical theory. It, too, is either incomplete or incorrect.

MITOCHONDRIAL THEORY

Mitochondria are the parts of the cells (organelles) that generate energy, so, as mentioned earlier, they are often called the powerhouses of the cells. It's a tough job, and mitochondria sustain a lot of molecular damage, so they must be recycled and replaced periodically to maintain peak efficiency. Cells undergo autophagy; mitochondria have a similar process of culling defective organelles for replacement, called *mitophagy*. The mitochondria contain their own DNA, which accumulates damage over time. The result is less-efficient mitochondria, which in turn produces more damage in a vicious cycle. Without adequate energy, cells may die, a manifestation of aging.

Muscle atrophy is related to high levels of mitochondrial damage.[13] But in comparing energy production in mitochondria in young and old people, little difference was found.[14] In mice, very high rates of mutation in mitochondrial DNA did not result in accelerated aging.[15]

> **Verdict:** This is an interesting theory, but the research is very preliminary and ongoing. Arguments can be made both for and against it.

HORMESIS

In 120 BC, Mithridates VI was heir to Pontus, a region in Asia Minor, or modern-day Turkey. During a banquet, his mother poisoned his father so that she could ascend the throne. Mithridates ran away and spent seven years in the wilderness. Paranoid about being poisoned, he chronically took small doses of poison to make himself immune. He returned as a man to overthrow his mother and claim the throne. He became a powerful king. During his reign, he opposed the Roman Empire but was unable to hold the Romans back. Before his capture, Mithridates decided to commit suicide by drinking poison. Despite taking large doses, "The Poison King" failed to die, and the exact cause of his death is still unknown.[16] What doesn't kill you may indeed make you stronger.

Hormesis is a phenomenon in which low doses of stressors that are normally toxic instead strengthen an organism and make it more resistant to higher doses of the same toxins or stressors. Fans of the movie *The Princess Bride* may remember that the hero, Westley, had taken small doses of iocane powder for years, which made him immune to its toxic effects. Thus, when Westley put the poison in both Vizzini's drink and his own, Westley was the only one to survive. This is hormesis.

Hormesis is not a theory of aging, but it has huge implications for other theories. The basic tenet of toxicology is "The dose makes the poison." Low doses of "toxin" may make you healthier.

Exercise and calorie restriction are examples of hormesis. Exercise, for example, puts stress on muscles causing the body to react by increasing muscular strength. Weight-bearing exercise puts stress on bones, causing the body to react by increasing bone strength. Being bedridden or going into zero gravity, as astronauts do, causes rapid weakening of muscles and bones.

Calorie restriction can be considered a stressor because it causes a rise in cortisol, commonly known as the stress hormone. This rise in cortisol increases the production of heat shock proteins (a family of proteins that help to stabilize new proteins or repair damaged ones) and resistance to subsequent stressors.[17] So, calorie restriction also satisfies the requirements of hormesis. Because both exercise and calorie restriction are forms of stress, they involve the production of free radicals.

Hormesis is not a rare phenomenon. Alcohol, for example, acts via hormesis. Moderate alcohol use is consistently associated with better health than complete abstention. But heavier drinkers have worse health and often develop liver disease. Exercise is well known to have beneficial health effects, but extreme exercise can worsen health by causing stress fractures. Even small doses of radiation can improve health, whereas large doses will kill you.[18]

Some of the beneficial effects of certain foods may be due to hormesis. Polyphenols are compounds in fruits and vegetables, as well as coffee, chocolate, and red wine, and they improve health, possibly in part by acting as low-dose toxins, thereby upregulating your body's natural endogenous antioxidant enzymes.

Why is hormesis important for aging? Other theories of aging presuppose that all damage is bad and accumulates over time. But the phenomenon of hormesis shows that the body has potent damage-repair capabilities that can be beneficial when activated. Take exercise as an example. Weight lifting causes microscopic tears in our muscles. That sounds pretty bad, but the process of repairing those muscles makes them stronger. Gravity puts stress on our bones. Weight-bearing exercise such as running causes microfractures of our bones. In the process of repair, our bones become stronger. The opposite situation exists in the zero gravity of outer space. Without the stress of gravity, bones become osteoporotic and weak.

Not all damage is bad—in fact, small doses of damage are good. What we are describing is a cycle of renewal. Hormesis allows the breakdown of tissue like muscle or bone that is then rebuilt to be better able to withstand the stresses placed upon it. Muscles and bones can grow stronger, but that growth can't happen without breakdown and repair.

Verdict: Hormesis has plenty of evidence that it's a true biological response to small doses of damage.

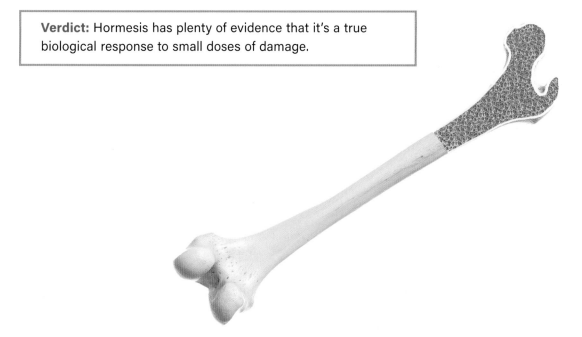

Growth Versus Longevity

Hormesis, like the disposable soma theory, suggests that there is a fundamental trade-off between growth and longevity. The larger and faster an organism grows, the faster it ages. Antagonistic pleiotropy may play a role in that some genes that are beneficial early in life may be detrimental later in life. When you compare life spans within the same species, such as in mice[19] and in dogs, smaller animals (the ones with less growth) live longer.[20] Women, on average smaller than men, also live longer. Among men, shorter men live longer.[21] Think about a person who is 100 years old. Do you imagine a muscular 6-foot-6-inch man, or do you picture a small woman?

Comparing across species, however, larger animals live longer. Elephants, for example, live longer than mice. But this difference can be explained by the slower development of larger animals.[22] The relative lack of predators for large animals has meant that evolution has favored slower growth and slower aging. Small animals that have fewer predators than other animals of the same size, such as bats, also live longer.

Aging isn't deliberately programmed, but the same physiologic mechanisms that drive growth also drive aging. Aging is simply the continuation of the same growth program, and it's driven by the same growth factors and nutrients. If you rev a car's engine, you can reach high speeds very quickly, but continuing to rev the engine results in burnout. It's the same essential program, but different time scales—short-term performance versus longevity. All the theories of aging point out this essential trade-off. This is powerful information because certain programs may be beneficial at certain times in our lives. During youth, for example, we need to grow. During middle and older age, however, this high growth program may cause premature aging, and it would be beneficial to slow growth. Because the foods we eat play a large role in this programming, we can make deliberate adjustments to our diet to preserve our life span as well as our "health span."

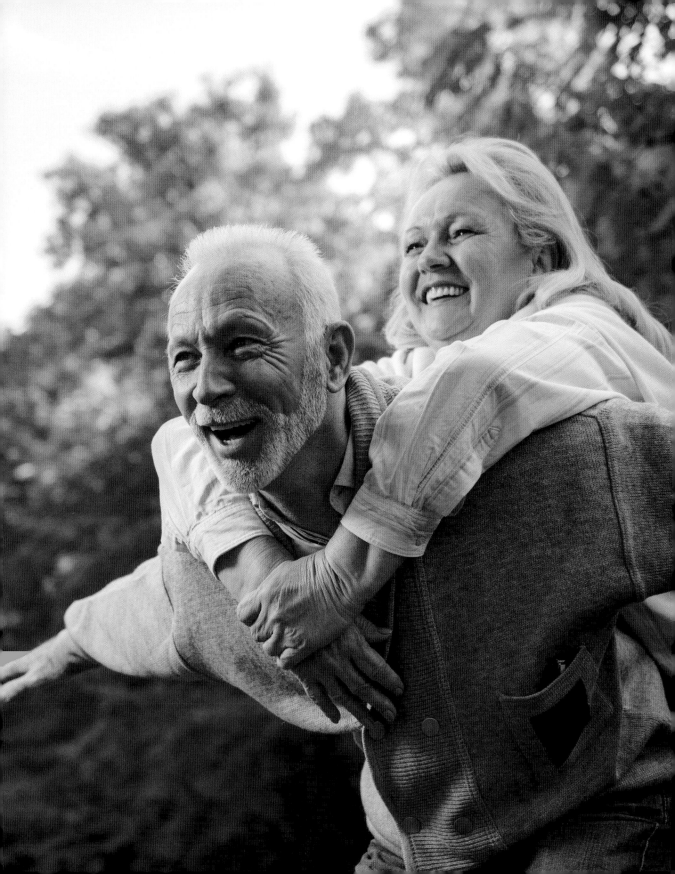

02

CALORIE RESTRICTION:

A DOUBLE-EDGED SWORD

The Calorie Restriction Society, which boasts more than 7,000 members, routinely restricts calories in the hope of living longer. Does that sound like a fantasy? Actually, among life-extension practices, perhaps the best described is calorie restriction, with animal studies dating back many decades. Calorie restriction (CR) with adequate nutrition is perhaps the most effective antiaging intervention currently known.[1]

Animal studies from as early as 1917 show that calorie restriction can prolong life. Restricting food intake in young female rats delays menopause, leaving them fertile far longer than normal. By 1935, researcher Clive McCay noted that reduced growth in white rats induced by calorie restriction resulted in increased longevity.[2] However, the animals must not be malnourished. Inadequate intake of essential vitamins and minerals causes many types of diseases, and malnourished mice generally do poorly and die young. Restricting energy (calories) while providing all the essential nutrients had the ability to extend life span, something previously unheard of.

Researchers have generally used a 40 percent calorie restriction, but even a 10 percent calorie restriction in rats gives nearly the same benefits.[3] A 10 percent calorie restriction increased life in these rats by about 15 percent, whereas animals restricted 40 percent lived about 20 percent longer. In 1942, researchers showed for the first time that calorie restriction in animals could prevent the development of cancer.[4] Controlled human studies are not available because they are virtually impossible to perform ethically. For the remainder of the book, we use the term *calorie restriction* with the implicit understanding that malnourishment must be avoided.

Calorie restriction extends the life span of every organism so far tested, including yeast, worms, flies, rodents, and monkeys. It also slows or even prevents age-related diseases, including dementia, diabetes, cardiovascular and coronary disease, neurodegenerative disorders, and several types of cancer. Researchers in 1946 insightfully noted that implementing a calorie-restricted diet in a plentiful food environment would be difficult or indeed impossible, as the ensuing decades would prove. Instead, they mused whether a more realistic form of calorie restriction could be implemented with a periodic fasting schedule. Rat experiments proved that this strategy was successful for life extension and cancer prevention.[5]

Extending this idea to humans, Ross, in 1959, noted that coronary heart disease is uncommon in nutritionally deprived communities.[6] In other words, populations that consume few calories seem to develop less heart disease. Researchers during this period also found a lesser effect of protein restriction on longevity. High casein (a form of dietary protein) in rat diets shortens life span.[7]

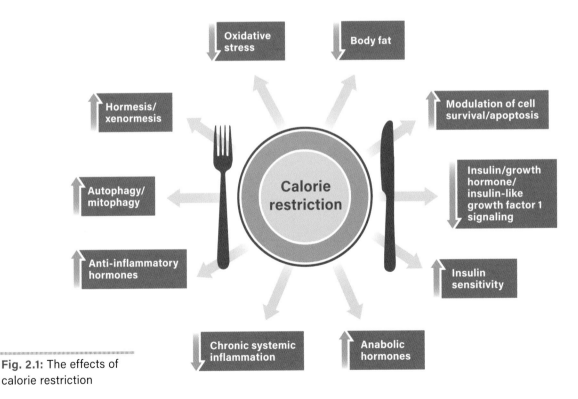

Fig. 2.1: The effects of calorie restriction

During the 1970s, Dr. Roy Walford at UCLA became the leading proponent of calorie restriction for longevity. He would later become the physician of Biosphere 2. This early 1990s experimental project was a self-contained greenhouse where eight "Terranauts" lived in a completely closed environment. They grew their own food and recycled their waste. However, they were unable to grow as much food as initially planned. Dr. Walford persuaded the other team members to finish their two-year mission while following a calorie-restricted diet. Unfortunately, things did not quite go as he had hoped. The Terranauts were likely not receiving adequate nutrition in addition to following a calorie-restricted diet. Dr. Walford lost 25 pounds from his already spare 145-pound frame and came out of Biosphere 2 considerably aged. He later developed Lou Gehrig's disease and died at age 79.

The 1980s saw the increasing acceptance of the calorie-restriction model and serious consideration of how to apply these animal studies to humans. More and more research publications are pushing the boundaries of knowledge of how calorie restriction can be a key component of longevity.

One of the most compelling examples of calorie restriction in prolonging human life span is in the Japanese prefecture of Okinawa. Traditionally, the Okinawan people follow a practice called *Hari Hachi Bu*, which is a sort of mindfulness eating. The Okinawans deliberately remind themselves to stop eating when they are 80 percent full, in effect self-imposing a 20 percent calorie restriction. There are a whopping four to five times more centenarians among their population than in most industrialized countries, and this trend has been associated with their low-calorie diets, which contain about 20 percent fewer calories than other Japanese people.[8] However, this impressive statistic doesn't extend to Okinawans who are younger than 65 years old, which might be linked to an increasingly Western-influenced diet that began to seep into their lifestyle starting in the 1960s. We talk more about the diet and life span of the Okinawans and other long-living cultures (in areas known as *Blue Zones*) in Chapter 12.

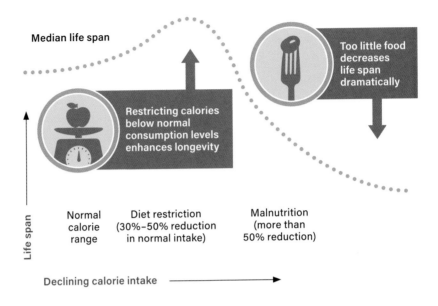

Fig. 2.2: Restricting calories enhances life span in animals

Calorie restriction is the only non-pharmacological method of consistently extending life span and protecting against many age-related diseases. When food is plentiful, animals, including humans, develop and grow, but they also age quickly. All animals have nutrient sensors, which are intricately linked to growth pathways. When animals detect a low availability of nutrients, growth is turned all the way down, which might induce longevity pathways in the essential balance between growth and longevity.[9] Of course, such restriction has its limits. Starvation and nutrient depletion cause death and disability. But calorie restriction with optimal nutrient intake is highly beneficial.

On its surface, this paradigm shift is fascinating. We often think about food as nourishment, so more should be better. But it's not. Instead, strategically depriving animals of food doesn't reduce life span; it extends it.

The Mechanisms of Calorie Restriction

Initially, the descriptions of life extension with calorie restriction seem radical, but studies have confirmed the relationship many times over in multiple species.[10]

Essentially, slower development and lower growth also resulted in longer life spans. Why? There are many potential mechanisms.

Low body fat is perhaps the most obvious effect of chronic calorie restriction in animals, but low visceral fat is of particular importance. High visceral fat, which is stored inside the abdomen and around major organs, poses a significant health risk to humans and is closely associated with decreased insulin sensitivity, obesity, type 2 diabetes, and atherosclerosis.

Mice genetically engineered to have very low body fat live longer. FIRKO (Fat Insulin Receptor Knock Out) mice have disrupted insulin receptors. Because insulin normally tells the body to gain fat, these genetically engineered mice cannot become obese, and they also live longer than unaltered mice. Both FIRKO and calorie-restricted mice have greatly reduced body fat, which suggests that less body fat might be the common denominator that extends life span.[11]

But that's not the whole story because being underweight or having lower-than-normal levels of fat also is associated with health risks. However, there's a large confounding factor here. Underweight people may have hidden illnesses, such as cancer, that cause the underweight condition, so it is unknown if deliberately lowering body fat below normal is healthy or harmful.

Chronic calorie restriction decreases the metabolic rate. If you eat fewer calories, your body responds by burning fewer calories. At first, this may not seem beneficial, but a lower metabolic rate correlates with less oxidative damage to DNA and therefore might affect aging.[12] Different animals have widely varying metabolic rates. In general, the higher the metabolic rate, the shorter the animal lives, possibly due to more free radical or oxidative damage.[13] If you are constantly revving your car's engine, it will go faster but burn out sooner. In humans, lower levels of free triiodothyronine (T3), a hormone important for metabolic rate, are associated with longer life.[14] Although calorie restriction can lower the overall metabolic rate, energy expenditure per gram of body weight may be higher.[15] Some reports have found healthy centenarians to have both greater muscle mass and a higher metabolic rate, both of which are correlated.[16]

Nutrient Sensors

The science of longevity always comes back to the competing interests of growth versus longevity. Higher growth generally results in lower longevity and vice versa. So, maximizing longevity often depends on reducing growth, and one of the ways we can influence this is through our nutrient sensors.

Primitive single-celled organisms live in a nutrient soup and can respond quickly to a decrease in nutrient availability by stopping growth. Yeast and bacteria, for example, go into a dormant (spore) form that can survive for thousands of years before becoming reanimated when water and nutrients are available. As we became complex multicellular creatures, we still needed to know whether nutrients were available. During a period of famine, we don't want to increase growth and metabolism, as this would hasten our demise. Having a lot of children during a famine might kill both mother and children, which is the reason that women without sufficient body fat stop ovulating. On the other hand, when food is plentiful, our bodies need to activate growth pathways to develop as quickly as possible. As the saying goes, make hay while the sun shines. Survival of all animals depends on both having nutrient sensors and linking them closely to growth pathways.

There are three known nutrient-sensing pathways: insulin, mTOR (mechanistic target of rapamycin), and AMPK (AMP-activated protein kinase). Extending longevity depends on decreasing growth and metabolism, which is best done by decreasing nutrient-sensing pathways by adjusting our diets. Reducing insulin (by lowering calories, but more specifically reducing refined grains and sugar), lowering mTOR (by reducing animal protein and using more plant proteins), and activating AMPK (by lowering calories) have all been linked to longevity.

INSULIN

The hormone insulin is the best known nutrient sensor. Food contains a mixture of the three macronutrients: carbohydrates, protein, and fat. When we eat, our bodies respond to these macronutrients by increasing the production of certain hormones. Insulin increases in response to eating carbohydrates and protein, but dietary fat does not stimulate insulin secretion. Insulin allows the cells of the body to use some ingested glucose for energy by acting on the protein GLUT4. As such, insulin fulfills the role of a nutrient sensor by signaling the availability of certain nutrients to the rest of the body.

But that's only one of insulin's roles. When insulin activates its receptor on the cell surface, it also activates the PI3K pathway, which results in protein synthesis and cell growth and division. This activation of PI3K happens simultaneously and automatically because these nutrient sensors link inextricably to growth pathways. Insulin plays a role in metabolism as well as in increasing growth, which is normally highly conducive to species survival because animals need to grow while food is available and stop growing when it is not.

Animal studies confirm that increasing nutrient availability decreases life span. Adding glucose to the food of the worm *C. elegans* shortens its life.[17] The high glucose stimulates insulin and promotes growth at the expense of a decreased life span. In humans, high insulin levels and insulin resistance, which are common in aging, have been consistently linked to increased risk of many age-related diseases, including cancer and heart disease.

During calorie restriction and fasting, blood glucose and insulin levels decline precipitously.[18] Lower insulin signaling decreases growth signaling but extends life span in several species of animals.[19] Decreasing carbohydrates in the diet is another natural method of decreasing insulin. Cynthia Kenyon, the scientist who discovered the roles of insulin and glucose in life extension, found the results so compelling that she went on a low-carbohydrate diet.[20] Increasing insulin sensitivity and lowering insulin levels may be an important mechanism in calorie restriction.

INSULIN-LIKE GROWTH FACTOR 1

A hormone closely related to insulin that plays a role in aging is insulin-like growth factor 1, or IGF-1. Growth hormone (GH), which is secreted by the pituitary gland, had always been assumed to be responsible for increasing growth in children. In the 1950s, Israeli endocrinologist Zvi Laron set up that country's first pediatric endocrine clinic. Among his first patients were several siblings with stunted growth. He assumed that they lacked GH, but when he measured their hormone levels, they were sky high. What was going on? Several decades of research would be needed before the answer was known.

Growth hormone acts on its cell receptor to produce IGF-1, which is the actual mediator of the growth effects. The children Laron encountered, who were suffering from what is now known as Laron dwarfism, had plenty of GH, but, because of a genetic defect in the receptor, they did not produce IGF-1. This lack of IGF-1 accounted for the children's short stature. Mystery solved. Later, though, a discovery in the Laron dwarfs would set the longevity world on fire in 2013.

In a remote corner of Ecuador lives a community of about 300 members known as the Laron dwarfs. A group of Spanish Jews in the fifteenth century fled the Inquisition, and genetic inbreeding led to this group of people who completely lack the hormone IGF-1. They grow to an average height of four feet but are otherwise normally formed. Dr. Guevara-Aguirre, a local physician, described and followed this community over several decades. He and his colleague, Dr. Valter Longo from the University of Southern California, made the startling discovery that these Laron dwarfs seemed to be completely immune to cancer![21] By comparison, unaffected relatives (those who do not have the syndrome) of these Laron dwarfs had a 20 percent rate of cancer.

Dr. Longo's interest in the longevity effect of less growth started in 2001 when he discovered that a long-lived yeast had the same type of growth pathway inhibition. Mice genetically deficient in growth hormone live 40 percent longer—the human equivalent of 110 years. Animals genetically engineered for high levels of growth hormone have short lives. Insulin and IGF-1 share many of the same features, and in some animals, the receptor is identical. This finding supports the notion that there's a fundamental trade-off between growth and longevity.

mTOR

Mammalian (or mechanistic) target of rapamycin (mTOR) is another important cellular nutrient sensor that is sensitive to dietary proteins and amino acids. When you eat protein, it gets broken down into its component amino acids for absorption by the intestines, and mTOR increases. Eating sufficient protein to obtain the necessary amino acids is important for overall health, but avoiding excessive mTOR is also important for life span extension.[22] Dietary protein restriction and fasting can decrease mTOR.

Like insulin, mTOR is a nutrient sensor, and its activation is inextricably linked to growth pathways. When you detect the availability of protein, your body goes into growth mode and begins producing new proteins. This is an example of antagonistic pleiotropy. In early life, mTOR promotes growth and development, but this mechanism harms us in later life by causing aging. Some of the benefits of protein restriction may be related to mTOR's effect on autophagy.

Autophagy is a cellular recycling process by which old proteins and subcellular organelles are broken down. This process provides energy and the amino acids necessary to rebuild new proteins to replace the old proteins, a key factor in cell maintenance. Autophagy is the critical first step for maintaining a cell in pristine condition, and aging is characterized by a decline in the rate of autophagy as damaged molecules accumulate in the cell and impede its function. In rats, there is as much as a six-fold difference between young and old animals.[23] Declining autophagy rates means that damaged cell components like lipid membranes and mitochondria hang around longer.

The most potent stimulus to turning off autophagy is mTOR. Even a little bit of dietary protein raises mTOR, turning off autophagy and the cellular renewal process. Fasting greatly increases the rate of autophagy and, in yeast, is essential to the life span–extending effects of calorie restriction.[24] Drugs that block mTOR, such as rapamycin, can extend life span in yeast, largely through its effect on autophagy.[25]

AMPK

The third nutrient sensor is known as AMP-activated protein kinase (AMPK). It acts as a sort of reverse fuel gauge of cellular energy stores. In your car, if you have lots of energy in the form of gasoline, the gauge reads high. In your cells, if you have lots of energy in the form of ATP (adenosine triphosphate), then AMPK is low.[26] Low cellular energy levels raise AMPK levels. Thus, AMPK acts as a sort of cellular fuel gauge but in reverse. Like mTOR and insulin, the nutrient sensor AMPK is linked to growth pathways. AMPK down-regulates synthesis of biological molecules, including those needed for growth (anabolism). Unlike insulin or mTOR, AMPK is not responsive to any specific dietary macronutrient but assesses the overall availability of cellular energy.

Substances that activate AMPK (mimicking low cellular energy stores) are known for promoting health. Examples include the diabetes drug metformin, resveratrol from grapes and red wine, epigallocatechin gallate (EGCG) from green tea and dark chocolate, capsaicin from peppers, curcumin from the spice turmeric, garlic, and the traditional Chinese medical herb berberine. Calorie restriction also activates AMPK, and this fact may be important to AMPK's effects on aging.[27]

AMPK enhances the uptake of glucose into muscle cells and increases the generation of mitochondria, leading to an increased capacity for burning fat. (See Figure 2.3.[28]) AMPK also increases autophagy, the important cellular self-cleansing process that rids cells of junk and recycles it, which we discuss in more detail later.

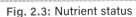

Fig. 2.3: Nutrient status

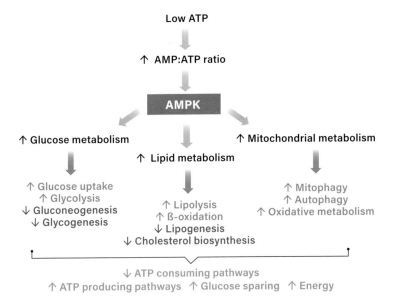

Intermittent Fasting

Intermittent fasting, which means going without food for some time, might have benefits for antiaging beyond simple calorie restriction. There are many different fasting regimens. One common form involves a sixteen-hour fast (including sleep time) and an eight-hour "feeding window." Some people practice alternate-day fasting, in which they eat little to no food on one day, and on the next day, eating is unrestricted.

Animals fed every other day behave physiologically like calorie-restricted animals, *even though they eat almost the same amount of food as fully fed animals.*[29] The animals that are fed every other day eat more on feeding days to compensate for their fasting days. This finding casts some doubt on whether fewer calories are essential to the life span extension. Although total calories are similar between calorie restriction and every-other-day fasting, the hormonal effects of fasting are very different. During fasting, all the nutrient sensor pathways are engaged—insulin and mTOR decrease while AMPK increases. Other hormones, known as the counterregulatory hormones, increase. These hormones include adrenaline, noradrenaline, and growth hormone. The increase in counterregulatory hormones has the effect of increasing energy and maintaining basal metabolic rate. These hormonal changes do not occur with simple chronic calorie reduction. The calories might be the same, but the physiologic effect is not. For example, reducing dietary fat reduces calories but not insulin or mTOR because the carbohydrate and protein intake may be unchanged.

Calorie-restricted (CR) animals are always hungry because of increased hunger hormone signaling.[30] Because hunger is such a fundamental instinct, it's virtually impossible to ignore hunger over the long term; hunger dooms many weight-loss programs to failure.

Fasting, on the other hand, often paradoxically decreases food cravings and hunger. Many patients note decreased hunger when using intermittent fasting for weight loss. They often comment that they think their stomach shrank when, in reality, hunger signaling decreased.

Rats and mice placed on an every-other-day feeding/fasting regimen live longer than fully fed animals. This result occurs without necessarily decreasing body weight, depending on the particular species of animal used.[31]

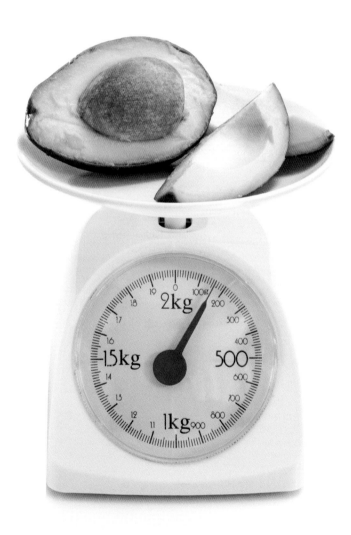

The Downsides of Calorie Restriction

Calorie restriction is useful only if you maintain adequate nutrition. You can take calorie restriction too far. Once a person falls below a certain threshold of body fat, there are concerns about decreased immune function,[32] low testosterone, feeling hunger, and feeling cold. These issues are not a major concern for the majority of Americans who are facing an obesity epidemic. Perhaps the most important problem with chronic calorie restriction is that it's difficult to maintain. You need to count *every* calorie scrupulously. You need to prepare all your food. You need to carefully calculate macronutrient ratios to make sure you get enough of each. You need to avoid junk food. These things aren't easy to do, and, in a lot of cases, it's not possible to do all of them all the time. Calorie restriction works on animals only when they are locked in cages. It doesn't work on most humans who have free will.

That's why scientists are so keen to discover the antiaging mechanisms behind calorie restriction. By understanding those mechanisms, we could mimic most of the benefits in a reasonable manner compatible with everyday life in twenty-first-century America.[33] There's good evidence that fewer calories may not lie at the heart of calorie restriction's benefits. Because the human body does not contain calorie receptors or calorie counters, the hormonal changes caused by dietary change must drive the benefits. Knowing these changes can lead us to natural "biohacks" (including changing dietary protein and consuming coffee, tea, and red wine, which we discuss further in subsequent chapters) that deliver all the same benefits.

03

mTOR AND LONGEVITY

In 1964, Georges Nógrády, a microbiologist at the University of Montreal, traveled to Easter Island, also known by its Polynesian name of Rapa Nui, to study the local population and collect soil samples. From those specimens, Dr. Suren Sehgal, who was working with a pharmaceutical company in Montreal, Canada, in 1972, isolated the bacterium *Streptomyces hygroscopicus.* This made a potent antifungal compound, which he isolated and named *rapamycin*, after the island of its origin. He hoped to make an antifungal cream for the topical treatment of athlete's foot, but the discovery turned out to be far more important.[1]

When Dr. Sehgal abruptly transferred to New Jersey, he couldn't bear the thought of destroying those samples. Instead, he wrapped some vials of rapamycin in heavy plastic, took them home, and stored them in his family freezer next to the ice cream with a label that said "DON'T EAT." Dr. Sehgal didn't resume work on rapamycin until 1987, when his company was bought out. Its antifungal properties turned out to be its least impressive feature.

Rapamycin suppresses the human immune system, so it's useful for treating eczema and as an antirejection medication in organ transplantation. By 1999, it was being used routinely in liver and kidney transplantation when scientists noted something odd. Most immune-suppressing drugs also increase the rates of cancer, but rapamycin did not. It *decreased* the risk of cancer! Rapamycin prevented cells from multiplying, and it displayed potent activity against solid tumors, both preventing new ones and curing pre-existing ones. Of course, this discovery was a breakthrough in cancer research.[2] Rapamycin derivatives also could slow the growth of cysts in the treatment of polycystic kidney disease.

More tantalizing was the realization that rapamycin might do something even more powerful—extend life span. Was the mythical fountain of youth sitting under the eternal gaze of Easter Island's famous Moai statues? This story is not science fiction; it's a tale in the thrilling world of real-life science.

How Does Rapamycin Work?

For decades after its discovery, what rapamycin did in the human body was a complete mystery. With rapamycin in hand, scientists could look for the targets within cells that interacted with this newly discovered drug. Like a homing beacon, rapamycin led them straight to a previously unknown biochemical pathway named (imaginatively) mammalian target of rapamycin (mTOR). That was astounding—the sort of thing that shouldn't happen. It was like suddenly discovering a new continent. Thousands of years of medical science had somehow missed this fundamental biological system. This nutrient-sensing pathway (mTOR) was so fundamental to life that it is conserved in animals from yeast all the way to humans. It is old in an evolutionary sense, older even than the much better-known insulin. The mTOR pathway is so critical that it is in virtually all life forms, rather than just mammals, so the name was changed to *mechanistic* target of rapamycin.

Nutrient sensors such as insulin and mTOR play a crucial role in an animal's survival by closely matching growth to nutrient availability. Think about a seed in the ground. When the proper conditions of available water, sunlight, and temperature exist, it will sprout. If the seed stays in a paper bag, it remains dormant. This ensures that the seed will not sprout into a hostile environment where it cannot survive. Animal cells are similar. If no nutrients are available to a cell, then it will not, and should not, grow. Instead, the cell slows growth and stays as "dormant" as possible. Nutrient sensors serve as the crucial link between nutrients and cell growth. If nutrients are available, then mTOR and insulin go up, and growth increases. If nutrients are not available, then mTOR and insulin go down, and growth slows. Growth depends on nutrients. And excessive growth may not be conducive to longevity.

The hormone insulin is sensitive to both dietary carbohydrates and protein, where mTOR is mostly stimulated by protein. mTOR plays a vital role in the health of mitochondria, the cell's energy generators. Like autophagy for mitochondria, low mTOR stimulates a process called *mitophagy*, where old, decrepit mitochondria are slated for breakdown. Once nutrients are again available, new mitochondria are produced. This renewal cycle ensures that the cells are maximally efficient during these feast/famine cycles—an important component of longevity and healthy aging.

The mTOR pathway is critical for regulating growth. There are two separate pathways, called the mechanistic target of rapamycin complex 1 and complex 2 (mTORC1 and mTORC2). Rapamycin, produced by bacteria to fight fungi, blocks mTOR and shuts down the fungi's growth pathways, putting them into a dormant state. In humans, slowing growth may prevent certain types of cancer, thus making it useful as a cancer medication. In the immune system, blocking mTOR could slow the growth of immune cells like the B and T cells, making it useful as an immune suppressant. In polycystic kidneys, blocking mTOR blocked the growth of new cysts. Rapamycin might also be useful for treating HIV infections, psoriasis, multiple sclerosis, and perhaps even Parkinson's disease.[3]

Many of these diseases happen to be associated with aging, which leads to one exciting proposition: Rapamycin is perhaps the most promising antiaging drug known. By slowing the growth mechanism of mTOR, it can not only prevent age-related diseases but also can slow down aging itself. Lower growth may equal more longevity. But is this being too optimistic?

An Antidote to Aging?

Since 1840, thanks to the Industrial Revolution, life expectancy has steadily increased around the world, especially in developed countries. The result is a fast-growing elderly population, which is estimated to double by 2050.[4] Along with the aging population come age-related diseases, including cancer, cardiovascular disease, type 2 diabetes, osteoporosis, and Alzheimer's.[5] Although lack of physical activity and smoking are important risk factors for heart disease, aging is by far the biggest risk factor.[6] It's pretty obvious when you think about it. Plenty of teenagers smoke and don't exercise, but they virtually never have heart attacks. On the other hand, there are plenty of 75-year-old people who don't smoke and do their exercise and still have heart attacks. Preventing such diseases goes hand in hand with slowing the aging process.

The discovery of rapamycin brought new life to the age-old dream of a life-extension pill. In animal models, rapamycin extends life span and its associated illnesses, although human studies are lacking. The first breakthrough came in 2006, when the life span of yeast more than doubled when the yeast was given rapamycin.[7] Subsequently, researchers found similar results in nematode worms (*C. elegans*),[8] who lived at least 20 percent longer on rapamycin, and then fruit flies, whose lives were extended by about 10 percent.[9]

Mice fed rapamycin lived 9 to 14 percent longer,[10] the first time a drug could extend the life of a mammal—with clear implications for humans. Currently, the only known way to extend the life of a rodent is through severe caloric restriction. Interestingly, this effect occurred no matter when the mouse started receiving the drug, whether the mouse was nine months (human equivalent thirty-five years) or twenty months (human equivalent sixty-five years).[11] To put this into perspective, a 10 percent increase in life span equates to an extra seven to eight years of life for a human being. Rapamycin improved heart function in middle-aged dogs,[12] marmosets,[13] and mice. It can block disease progression in mouse models of Alzheimer's disease[14] by increasing neuronal autophagy. When mice receive rapamycin early, it prevents age-related learning and memory deficits in mice.[15] Giving rapamycin to aging obese rats can reduce appetite and body fat.[16] Other benefits indicated by animal studies include potential prevention of age-related retinopathy (the most common cause of blindness in Western countries)[17] and improvements in depression and anxiety, autism, and autoimmune disorders.[18]

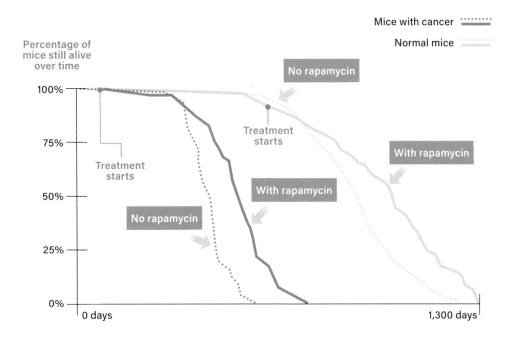

Mice with cancer

Normal mice

Percentage of mice still alive over time

No rapamycin

Treatment starts

With rapamycin

100%

75%

Treatment starts

50%

With rapamycin

No rapamycin

25%

0%

0 days   1,300 days

Graphic data by Bloomberg Businessweek
Data for female mice shown, data NIH 2009, Aging 2013

Fig. 3.1: The effect of rapamycin on the life span of mice

But what about the effect on humans? The story is a little more complicated. All drugs have side effects, and rapamycin is no exception. Suppressing the immune system increases the risk of infections. Growth-suppressing effects may increase lung toxicity, ulceration of the mouth, diabetes, and hair loss.[19] Consequently, by taking rapamycin, you might extend your life span or cut it short from an infection.[20] The optimal dosing schedule is still unknown because almost all human studies have been done in specific disease conditions, such as cancer, post-transplant, or polycystic kidney disease. On the other hand, long-term rapamycin treatment may cause significant metabolic side effects.[21]

The chronic use of rapamycin can cause insulin resistance and raise cholesterol and triglyceride levels.[22] But intermittent use of rapamycin might lower the incidence of these side effects, which could help realize its full potential. Shorter-term, intermittent treatment could still extend life span and reduce disease.[23] Rapamycin treatment delivered just once every five days showed significant impact on T-cells without affecting glucose tolerance.[24] This intermittent, rather than constant, blockage of mTOR is likely *crucial* because our natural diets alternate periods of feasting and fasting. Insulin and mTOR should naturally be periodically cycling between high and low levels rather than staying high or low constantly. It is in the balance of growth and longevity that we find optimal health.

For longevity, lower doses of rapamycin might be more effective. With age, mTOR might be overactive, driving the body's growth pathways more than the maintenance pathways. Turning down the mTOR activity might help organs, including the immune system.[25] High mTOR during childhood and youth is normal because growth is more important than longevity during this phase of life.

The nutrient sensor AMPK goes in the opposite direction of insulin and mTOR, like a seesaw (see Figures 3.2 and 3.3). If nutrients are available, mTOR, insulin, and IGF-1 are high, and AMPK is low, which favors growth and reproduction. When nutrients are not available, mTOR, insulin, and IGF-1 are low, and AMPK is high. The cells have low energy and favor maintenance, repair, and survival. Health lies in the balance. Sometimes we need growth, and other times we need maintenance and repair. So the ideal schedule is to cycle these states regularly, something that is easier with intermittent fasting. Certain drugs and foods can also influence these levels.

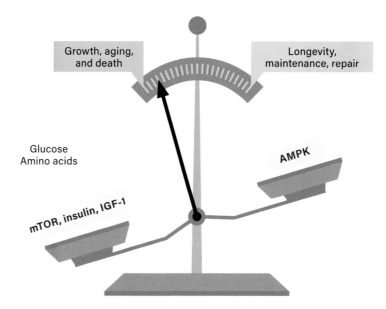

Fig. 3.2: High nutrient availability

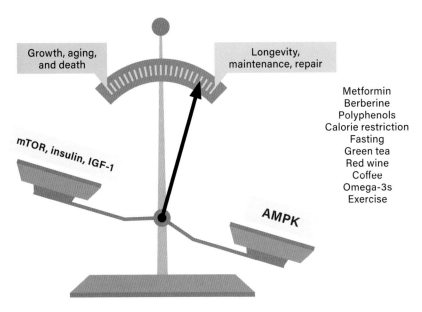

When a person follows a plan of intermittent fasting, he restricts calorie intake within a defined period. For example, he might eat during eight hours of each day and fast for the remaining sixteen hours. This pattern naturally cycles the body through both high and low nutrient availability and might maximize both growth and longevity pathways. Since as early as the 1940s, we've known that intermittent fasting makes rats live longer.[26] Recent studies in humans show that intermittent fasting increases SIRT1 and SIRT3, mitochondrial proteins that can promote longevity in response to oxidative stress.

Ultimately, to slow aging and reduce age-related diseases without the downsides of rapamycin, we need to target the mTOR pathway in a different but more natural way—through our diets. Specifically, we need to talk more about the main stimulus to mTOR: dietary protein.

Protein Restriction, IGF-1, and mTOR

Since the 1960s, we've gone from discussing foods to discussing *macronutrients*, the three main components of food: proteins, fats, and carbohydrates. Reducing dietary fat and cholesterol to prevent heart disease has been a key public health message. This recommendation turned out to be far too simplistic, with recent studies showing that dietary saturated fat and cholesterol have little effect on heart disease risk.[27] The Dietary Guidelines for Americans encouraged eating more carbohydrates, like white bread and pasta, and by the late-1970s, the obesity epidemic began. Some forty years later, it continues to accelerate. Currently, about 70 percent of Americans are overweight or obese. Much ink has been spilled on the various pitfalls of eating too much or too little fat and carbohydrates, but protein is largely forgotten. Should we eat more or less? How much is too much? How much is too little? What types of protein are best? These are all critical questions for our health.

Most of our bodies' structural systems, such as skeletal muscle, bone, and organs, are largely made up of proteins. The enzymes and hormones that control our biochemistry are proteins, too. There are an estimated 250,000 to 1 million different types of protein molecules in the human body.[28] The building blocks to make all the necessary proteins are called *amino acids*, and they come mostly from our diet. The body digests and absorbs protein from food as amino acids, and our bodies reassemble these into new proteins necessary for normal, healthy functioning.

Each protein is made by stringing amino acids together in a specific sequence, so each protein has a unique structure and function. All of the thousands of different proteins in the human body are made by only twenty amino acids, just as the twenty-six letters of the alphabet can be arranged to make millions of different words.

Of the twenty amino acids, eleven are nonessential because humans can synthesize them. The other nine are called essential amino acids because humans must obtain them from food. Being deficient in even one essential amino acid forces the body to break down its own proteins to get the required amino acid. Prolonged deficiency results in illness or even death. The body stores very little amino acids, so you must eat a diet that supplies adequate amounts of essential amino acids. If you eat more amino acids than necessary, the body may use them as a source of energy by transforming them into glucose via a process known as *gluconeogenesis.*

Consuming adequate amounts of protein is important for maintaining muscle mass. In the modern Western world, the elderly are more susceptible to excessive muscle loss known as *sarcopenia.* Loss of muscle strength may cause falls, broken bones, and an inability to carry out the activities of daily living, leading to institutionalization. Extreme cases of protein deficiency cause a disease known as *kwashiorkor*, which is characterized by a large belly and thin extremities. But the possibility that excess protein could also be a problem has been largely ignored, as we'll discuss later.

Protein-rich animal foods (meat or eggs) are much more expensive than carbohydrate-rich foods (bread or rice). Affluent Western nations tend to eat more protein, which increases the risk of overconsumption and lowers the risk of protein deficiency. Plant proteins differ from animal protein in their amino acid composition, which has important consequences for health and disease. Different stages of life have different protein demands. Fine-tuning protein intake can slow aging, prevent illness, and increase strength.

The recommended daily allowance (RDA) of protein as set by the U.S. government is 0.8 gram per kilogram of body weight; that's considered a minimum. At least half of American men consume more than 1.34 grams per kilogram of body weight. Vegetarians generally consume less protein, about 0.75 gram per kilogram on average, and have significantly lower IGF-1 levels. Again, this is likely a good thing because IGF-1 stimulates growth, which may reduce longevity. The beneficial effects of calorie restriction, despite its name and method, may not depend on eating fewer calories at all.[29] Restricting protein without lowering calories can promote health and longevity, too.[30]

Protein restriction, which reduces IGF-1 and mTOR, might be responsible for the majority of the benefits of calorie reduction.[31] Restricting calories without restricting protein does not lower IGF-1 levels, which might promote growth, but not longevity. Lowering protein reduces IGF-1 by 25 percent, which may be a large component of "anticancer and anti-aging dietary interventions."[32] But how much protein we need depends on our circumstances. Athletes need more protein than other people, and cutting down on protein too much may be harmful. The key is to find the balance between too much protein and too little—a topic we discuss in Chapter 6.

Other Ways to Reduce mTOR

Aside from diet, there are other ways to reduce mTOR. Rapamycin is one example of a drug known to block mTOR. Aspirin, curcumin, and green tea extract seem to be mTOR inhibitors and extend life span. Epigallocatechin 3-gallate (EGCG), which is in green tea, might protect against cancer, reduce weight, and stimulate fat loss.[33] Polyphenols are naturally occurring antioxidants found in plants that may slow aging by targeting the mTOR and AMPK pathways.[34] Allspice, hibiscus, curcumin, and pomegranate are rich in polyphenols and may inhibit cancer by suppressing mTOR.[35] The polyphenol from red wine, resveratrol, generated much initial scientific excitement,[36] but resveratrol supplements showed disappointing results that didn't live up to the hype.

The type 2 diabetes drug metformin is derived from a medicinal plant that humans have used for hundreds of years. It lowers glucose and insulin, which may be due to its ability to stimulate AMPK and inhibit mTOR.[37] This reason might be why metformin, like rapamycin, is associated with a lower risk of cancer.[38] Most intriguingly, though, diabetics who take metformin appear to live longer than nondiabetics who do not.[39]

Growth Versus Longevity

Fast growth allows animals to mature quickly and have children, which propagates their genes into the next generation. High growth improves the odds of animals reproducing, but that fast growth rate may increase aging. To the gene, however, faster aging is irrelevant, because aging and death generally occur long after reproduction. If the animal has offspring, the gene will survive even after the individual animal perishes. Evolution requires constant renewal, and longevity is a deterrent to this goal, so it can be considered somewhat "unnatural." The gene "rejuvenates" itself by letting an older individual die and renewing itself in that person's children.

> *Evolution favors constant renewal over longevity.*

To slow aging, we must counteract our embedded evolutionary heritage. In the battle between growth and longevity, besides the nutrient sensors, it is worth considering growth hormone (GH) and the related insulin-like growth factor 1 (IGF-1).

Several decades ago, before the concept of growth versus longevity was well known, some researchers had what seemed like a brilliant idea. The genes for GH had been sequenced, and it had just become possible to produce human GH relatively easily with recombinant DNA technology. Before that, injectable GH to treat the relatively rare disease of GH deficiency was produced by grinding up the pituitary gland of cadavers (dead bodies) and purifying the GH. The process was difficult, expensive, and rather gross. Now that pure GH was easily producible, perhaps it could be used as an antiaging treatment to rejuvenate the bodies of older adults.

A 1990 study showed that injecting growth hormone in older people caused them to lose body fat, gain muscle, and have improved energy and sex drive.[40] Sounds pretty great, right? But there was a dark side. The injections also promoted cancer, heart failure, and diabetes, demonstrating that growth hormone potently *promotes* aging. People who suffer from excessive growth hormone keep growing and die early—growth versus longevity.

Growth hormone is the main stimulant to IGF-1. Both are highest in growing children and adolescents and decline into adulthood and old age, reflecting the different priorities of each stage of life. Childhood and early adulthood are periods in which growth is the priority, so GH and IGF-1 are high. Later in life, though, these high levels of GH and IGF-1 become detrimental to longevity. Studies of centenarians have revealed that less growth hormone and IGF-1 are associated with better health and longer life.

Interestingly, though, GH levels are significantly elevated during fasting. Huh? Why would the body increase GH when no nutrients are available? The reason GH increases during fasting is that fasting induces a state of "GH resistance." This is caused by activation of fibroblast growth factor 21 (FGF-21), which reduces IGF-1 and increases liver expression of IGF-1 binding protein 1 to blunt GH signaling.[41] Thus, while GH may be higher during fasting, there is actually less growth and more repair.

Dietary protein increases levels of both GH and IGF-1, which may be good or bad, depending on your stage in life. When we are young, protein helps us mature, ensures that all systems are healthy and strong, and readies us for conceiving, bearing, and caring for children. In an adult, too much protein might promote cancer, heart disease, and other ills of aging. Considered in this new light, many of the diseases that affect adults are diseases of "too much growth."

For example, atherosclerosis is the underlying process of "hardening of the arteries" that causes heart attacks and strokes. Initially thought to be a disease of cholesterol blocking the arteries, it is now known to be a disease of excessive smooth muscle proliferation and inflammation that blocks the arteries. "Too much growth" in the blood vessels leads to blockages. Cancer is a disease of "too much growth" that is uncontrolled. Obesity, with its related metabolic diseases, is a disease of "too much growth."

Reining in this epidemic of "too much growth" depends on decreasing growth pathways. The key to reaping the antiaging, antidisease benefits of calorie restriction is getting the right amount and balance of dietary protein appropriate to your stage of life and lifestyle.

It All Comes Down to Protein

Longevity is not just about calories.[42] (Is it ever?!) Protein restriction plays a large role in extending life span[43] by slowing growth (and aging). Manipulation of dietary protein is potentially easier than restricting calories or fasting, but it has similar benefits.[44] Even as early as the 1930s, animal studies showed that protein restriction can double life span.[45] Mice live longest with a diet of just 5 percent protein; at that level, they also have lower rates of cancer[46] and lower cholesterol.[47] One specific essential amino acid, methionine, may be especially important.[48] Plant-based diets are not only lower in protein but often low in methionine specifically.

Low-protein diets might reduce cancer and mortality in humans.[49] Customizing our diets—specifically our protein intake—could stave off disease and promote longer life. The key to longevity might already be in your hands. It's not a magical berry from a far-off land. It's not even a stringent low-calorie diet. It starts with simply optimizing your protein intake.

Is Aging Just a Program We Can Update?

The master program that drives growth, mTOR, doesn't magically turn off when we're older. It also drives aging. This growth versus longevity paradox means that the mTOR so necessary for early life may also lead to early death. But perhaps there are ways to reprogram our cells to slow aging.[50] Perhaps all we need is an update in our software.

04
DIETARY PROTEIN

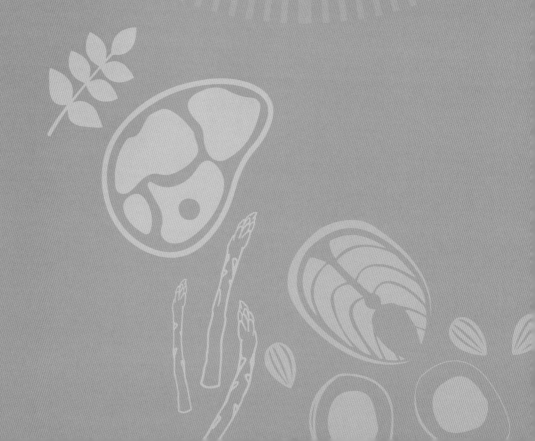

Restricting dietary protein might promote longevity, but if taken too far, it will also inhibit normal growth and cause malnutrition. Protein deficiency can occur in isolation, or it can occur as part of a general lack of food. Overall starvation, with not only protein deficiency but also fat deficiency, is called *marasmus.* People become skeletally thin, with no body fat and wasting of muscle. In other situations, people get sufficient calories but very little protein.

This issue of getting enough calories without enough protein typically occurs in children in the war-torn nations of sub-Saharan Africa that rely on food aid. These people receive mostly refined carbohydrates (which are cheap) but almost no protein (which is expensive). Food donation by First World countries typically is refined carbohydrates (sugar, flour, rice, corn), which provide calories at a fraction of the cost of protein and, importantly, do not require refrigeration during the long trip. The 1970s and 1980s saw many cases of isolated protein deficiency called *kwashiorkor.* African children had swollen feet, thin arms and legs (due to loss of muscle), hair loss, poor immune function, and a swollen fatty liver (due to excess carbohydrates).

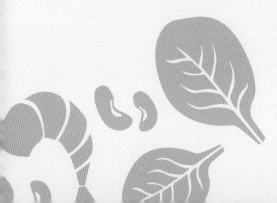

Kwashiorkor affects mostly children because of the importance of dietary protein for proper growth in infancy and childhood. Adults may break down their own protein and recycle the amino acids, but children must eat sufficient protein to grow. In developed nations, kwashiorkor is virtually absent, so we rarely see severe protein deficiency in these areas.

As humans move into middle age, growth is no longer necessary, and it's possibly detrimental to longevity. Low protein intake is associated with a reduction in IGF-1, as well as a reduction in cancer and overall mortality in people 65 or younger, but not in those older than 65.[1]

As we age (especially as we pass the age of 65), too little protein can be detrimental, as we typically lose muscle over time. Of all human tissue, muscle burns the most energy. Muscle wasting, or atrophy, can start at as early as 30 years of age. On average, people lose 10 percent of their muscle mass per decade of life. By age 80, the typical person may have lost a full 50 percent of muscle mass. (See Figure 4.1.) Loss of muscle, known as *sarcopenia,* has dire consequences, including the inability to perform simple tasks of daily living, such as getting out of a chair or even standing. Lack of exercise likely plays a large role in sarcopenia, as studies of traditional societies with an active lifestyle have shown that those individuals maintain muscle mass and strength. However, in Western societies, we tend to become more sedentary with age, and we might need more protein due to a phenomenon known as *anabolic resistance.*

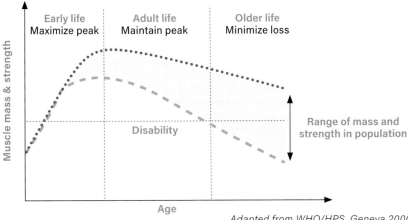

Fig. 4.1: Muscle mass and aging

Anabolic resistance is the phenomenon in which sufficient dietary protein, and particularly the amino acid leucine, results in less muscle growth (anabolism) in older people than in the young. Most tissues of the body, including muscle and bone, are in a constant state of breakdown and repair. For example, cells called *osteoclasts* break down bone tissue, whereas other cells called *osteoblasts* lay down new bone. Sometimes this renewal cycle moves slowly, and sometimes it can be accelerated, as with fasting.

Fasting decreases insulin and mTOR and activates the breakdown of protein. The body has some amino acids in the bloodstream at all times, and when eating is resumed, the high growth hormone levels help rebuild muscle to replace that which was lost. If you are doing exercise, then the muscle is rebuilt to carry more weight. We should emphasize that this cycle involves small amounts of muscle. You are not in danger of losing much, if any, muscle mass through periodic short-term (i.e., 24-hour) fasting. This renewal cycle is similar to autophagy, which happens at a subcellular level and involves organelles and mitochondria. In older people, anabolic resistance means more protein is necessary for this cycle of muscle breakdown and growth. Eating more protein can help older people overcome this phenomenon.

Restricting calories is not the same as restricting protein. Members of the Calorie Restriction Society (CRS), which was founded in 1993, deliberately restrict calories for longevity and wellness. They don't follow a low-protein diet, however. Scientific studies found their protein intake rather high at 1.7 grams per kilogram of body weight per day compared to 1.2 grams on a typical Western diet and only 0.8 gram on a vegan diet. The CRS group's IGF-1 levels were not much different compared to a standard Western diet.[2] Only the vegan group showed decreased IGF-1. When some of the CRS group decreased their protein intake to 0.95 gram, their IGF-1 levels dropped by 22 percent and measured only slightly higher than the vegan group. Protein intake is critically important for IGF-1 levels in humans, despite calorie restriction. The vegan group in the study consumed more calories but less protein than the CRS group. And the protein they consumed was only plant protein. So lowering IGF-1 seems to have more to do with protein restriction than calorie restriction.

While the decrease in IGF-1 that's observed with lower protein intake appears encouraging, the relation between IGF-1 and longevity is still unproven. Yet the Laron dwarfs we mentioned in Chapter 2 are an example of the importance of low IGF-1 levels for cancer and other diseases of aging.

Aging and Amino Acids

Proteins are composed of individual amino acids, and certain amino acids are worth discussing in more detail.

CYSTEINE The nonessential amino acid cysteine is crucial for the formation of glutathione (the body's internal antioxidant), which tends to decline with age. When the body is depleted of glutathione, it's less able to handle oxidative stress, and eating more cysteine may help solve this problem. The close association among aging, oxidative stress, and cysteine has even led some scientists to deem aging a "cysteine deficiency syndrome"; ensuring an adequate supply of cysteine might go a long way toward ameliorating the maladies of aging. Cysteine is in most high-protein foods; for example, meat, dairy, onions, broccoli, Brussels sprouts, and oats are high in cysteine.

LEUCINE The amino acid leucine plays a key role as a signaling molecule in muscle growth and critical processes such as autophagy. Together, leucine, isoleucine, and valine are known as branched-chain amino acids (BCAAs). All three BCAAs are essential amino acids and are important for building muscle.

Specific situations in which more BCAAs are useful include those situations in which a great deal of growth is desired. Bodybuilders often take whey supplements, which contain large amounts of leucine. Burn victims often lose massive amounts of protein, and supplementing with leucine might be a useful strategy to increase growth of new tissue.[3] Whey also can be useful for the elderly and ill due to its growth-promoting effects on mTOR.

METHIONINE

The amino acid methionine is one of the nine essential amino acids. Restricting methionine, even without overall caloric restriction, has the astounding ability to increase life span in certain species, including the fruit fly and mouse.[4] Methionine-restricted animals have less body fat and better insulin sensitivity and metabolism. Methionine is in meat, eggs, fish, some nuts, seeds, and cereal grains. Fruits and vegetables, including legumes, although otherwise protein dense, contain little methionine. This offers the tantalizing possibility that dietary changes could extend human life span. However, since methionine is an essential amino acid, you cannot eliminate it from the diet entirely. (Remember, essential amino acids are the type of amino acids that your body cannot make.)

GLYCINE

Glycine is the most important nonessential amino acid. It represents 11.5 percent of the total amino acids in the body and is an important precursor for vital proteins such creatine (in muscle), glutathione (an antioxidant), and heme (in blood). Glycine supplementation appears to be particularly unique, as it may afford protection against dietary fructose in animal models.[5] And considering that the typical American consumes around 50 pounds of fructose per year, the protective potential of glycine supplementation is advantageous.

Glycine is also important for the skin and joints. Gelatin, such as that found in Jell-O brand desserts, is a particularly rich source of glycine. It is produced by boiling the bones and skins of cows and pigs. Bone broth is also a good dietary source of glycine. Horses' hooves, despite the popular myth, do not contain sufficient collagen, the connective tissue around the joints, to be used in the production of gelatin. In Asia, tendons, high in glycine, are prized delicacies.

Methionine lowers glycine levels by reducing absorption and increasing excretion. Some of the benefits of methionine restriction might be due to higher glycine levels. Glycine might mimic methionine restriction by changing amino acid metabolism. Increasing the glycine content of diets might offer an easy way to obtain the effects of methionine restriction and, thus, life extension.

All these amino acids play a role in normal human metabolism. We must get enough protein to stay healthy, but the million-dollar question is how much protein is too little, and how much protein is too much?

How Much Protein Is Too Little?

The Institute of Medicine of the National Academy of Sciences set the Recommended Daily Allowance (RDA) for protein to be 0.8 gram per kilogram of body weight. For the average man, that amounts to about 56 grams of protein a day; for the average woman, it's about 46 grams. This is not the same as 46 to 56 grams of meat, because protein makes up only about 16 to 25 percent of the weight of meat, depending upon the type and the leanness. If you eat 56 grams of steak, you're not getting a full 56 grams of protein. You require about six times more by weight (approximately) to offset the portion of the steak that's not protein. How did the Institute of Medicine come up with this RDA of 0.8?

You can estimate the amount of protein you need from the amount your body loses on a daily basis, assuming you are maintaining weight rather than losing or gaining it. Protein losses can be measured by checking nitrogen losses in the urine and stool. Carbohydrates and fat are composed mainly of carbon and hydrogen, whereas protein is the major source of nitrogen in the body. In 1985, the World Health Organization found that daily losses of protein averaged 0.61 gram per kilogram per day. Presumably, then, a person's diet should replace (roughly) this 0.61 gram per kilogram per day that's lost. This average is for normal healthy people, not for people who are losing muscle or otherwise are sick.

To build in a margin of safety against protein deficiency, the World Health Organization added 25 percent (two standard deviations) more than the 0.61 gram per kilogram per day value, which is approximately 0.8 gram per kilogram per day. Based on the original calculations, 97.5 percent of the healthy general population was eating less than 0.8 gram per kilogram per day of amino acids. This value is not a low standard. This is a very high standard of sufficient protein intake, *and the value was calculated on the assumption that excess dietary protein is not dangerous*.

Even at this high level, the average man still required only 56 grams of protein and the average woman only 46 grams. For reference, the USDA in 1985 determined that in the United States, 14 to 18 percent of calories came from protein, and the average consumption was 90 to 110 grams per day for men and 70 grams per day for women. Americans, being one of the wealthiest populations on Earth, were eating much more protein than the average inhabitants of this planet. The average American male was eating twice the recommended daily amount, which itself is already a high estimate of our actual needs. This happens day after day. Week after week. Year after year.

Furthermore, in adults, our bodies continuously degrade and resynthesize intrinsic body proteins. Old proteins are broken down, and the amino acids are reabsorbed to be built into new proteins. The amount of turnover is several times larger than the amount of amino acids we eat daily. However, some amino acids do get lost in the process, predominantly in the stool and urine. During periods of low protein intake, the amount of nitrogen lost in the stool and urine can drop to a very low level, which explains how adults in sub-Saharan Africa largely avoided kwashiorkor despite extremely low protein intake. Their bodies were recycling their own amino acids to build new proteins. So, the lower limit of protein needed to maintain health is largely still unknown, but it might be far lower than 0.61 gram per kilogram per day.

Protein intake is best calculated using grams per kilogram of lean body mass because fat tissue requires little to no protein for maintenance. Online body fat calculators can provide a reasonable estimate of your lean body mass using gender, weight, and waist circumference.[6] For example, if someone weighs 200 pounds and has 25 percent body fat, that would imply 75 percent lean mass. Total lean mass is then simply calculated like so:

<u>200 pounds x 0.75 = 150 pounds (68 kilograms) of lean mass</u>

If that person ate 68 grams of protein per day, he would consume 1.0 gram per kilogram of lean mass.

These recommendations differ due to individual differences and the type of protein consumed. Animal protein is a more digestible and complete source of protein, so we likely require less. We likely require more plant proteins (such as from soy or legumes) because of its lower absorption (bioavailability).

So, should you worry about protein deficiency? Not really. In the United States, the average person eats approximately twice the RDA, which itself is designed to be higher than a healthy person needs. If we start seeing a North American outbreak of kwashiorkor, we'll start worrying. So, this brings us to the opposite question.

How Much Protein Is Too Much?

Excess protein, beyond what you need to maintain structural tissues such as muscle, is metabolized for energy or stored as glycogen or fat. Like excess carbohydrate or sugar, excess protein might lead to metabolic problems like obesity and type 2 diabetes. A low-carbohydrate diet might resolve many of these problems, such as insulin resistance and obesity, by allowing fat to be used preferentially as an energy source; low-protein diets might be beneficial in the same way.[7]

The answer is highly dependent on the situation. If you are trying to build muscle, as in body building, you need to eat more protein to sustain muscle growth. Pregnancy, breastfeeding, and typical growth in children are situations in which growth is normal, and more protein is required.

On the other hand, if you are trying to lose weight, then you should eat less protein than the 0.61 gram per kilogram per day estimate. Overweight and obese people not only have more body fat but also an estimated 20 to 50 percent more protein than a lean person. Different types of protein loss need to happen along with fat loss—skin, connective tissue, capillaries, blood vessels, and so on. All this protein needs to be catabolized (burned up and not replaced). You often hear about how surgeons must remove 20 to 30 pounds of excess skin and tissue after significant weight loss. Yes, that's all protein that should have been catabolized.

Some people argue that protein builds muscle. Hmm. Eating protein without exercise builds muscle? Right. Dream on. If that were true, we would not have an obesity epidemic; we'd have a muscle epidemic. Americans eat more protein than most of the rest of the world, and the cover of *Time* magazine has never posed the question, "Is America too muscular?" Although adequate protein is necessary for good health, more is not always better. Some of the antiaging benefits of calorie restriction are due to less protein but likely also less refined carbohydrates. However, too little protein may lead to sarcopenia and frailty. Longevity requires a happy medium.

Dietary protein, through mTOR, stops autophagy, which declines with age; the result is the accumulation of damaged molecules.[8] The amino acid leucine, which is in virtually all proteins, is a key regulator of autophagy; when leucine levels in the bloodstream rise, autophagy quickly drops, and vice versa. Conversely, intermittent fasting promotes autophagy.

The role of leucine means that you don't need to lower your protein intake much, if at all, to get the benefits of increased autophagy (although you might need to lower overall protein to get the benefits of reduced IGF-1). Decreased meal frequency, such as eating only once a day or eating only during a restricted feeding "window," such as an eight-hour period daily, may activate autophagy without reducing calories or protein overall.

Longer periods of fasting, coupled with lower protein intake, have a pronounced antiaging effect through the renewal of immune system cells.[9] Other diets that mimic fasting might have some benefit, too.[10]

Lower protein intake over a period of hours to days can have many benefits. Resuming normal protein intake then stimulates muscle to renew itself. This system of protein cycling could promote life extension while preventing muscle loss.

Based on these physiologic principles, a low-carbohydrate, adequate-protein diet would produce many of the benefits of calorie restriction. Carbohydrates, particularly refined carbs, stimulate both insulin and mTOR, which turns off autophagy. A diet low in carbohydrates and only moderate in protein would involve eating lots of natural fats, which are not to be feared. Dietary fat does not stimulate insulin, mTOR, or IGF-1. Indeed, early research confirmed that a high-fat, adequate protein, low-carb diet dramatically improved biomarkers of aging, such as improvements in body weight, leptin, fasting glucose, insulin, and triglycerides.[11] As a side benefit, subjects lost an average of 8 kilograms (17.6 pounds) in body weight. Specific restriction of the dietary amino acid methionine decreased mitochondrial damage. The subjects were counseled to limit their protein intake to 1.0 gram per kilogram of lean body mass; those subjects who exercised were told to increase the quantity to 1.25 grams. Lose weight and increase longevity? Sounds like a plan.

05

PLANT VERSUS ANIMAL PROTEIN

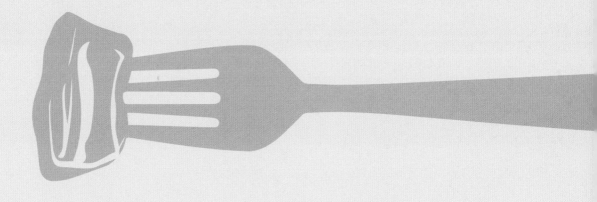

Jordan Peterson, a professor at the University of Toronto and bestselling author, and his daughter, Mikhaila, have both followed in recent years a carnivorous diet, consisting of meat, salt, and little else. Mikhaila had been diagnosed with juvenile rheumatoid arthritis, depression, and idiopathic hypersomnia. All that disappeared when she switched to eating meat only. They eat 100 percent animal foods. Vegans, on the other hand, eat no animal products, so they eat 100 percent plant foods. Major food chains have added vegan choices including meatless burgers. Guinness, the famous Irish beer, stopped using fish bladders in its brewing process after more than 200 years. According to the newspaper the *Guardian*, we are witnessing the "unstoppable rise of veganism: how a fringe movement went mainstream."[1] Members of each group feel terrific on either all plant or all animal foods. Who is correct? Which proteins are optimal for health—animal or plant? What does the science tell us?

We often associate the word *protein* with animal foods. However, vegetables also contain protein in varying amounts. Tofu, chickpeas, lentils, beans, wheat (gluten is a protein), nuts, and seeds are sources of plant proteins. We rarely see serious protein deficiency in North America, except perhaps in alcoholics. So, a largely vegetarian diet is not necessarily deficient in protein. Instead, the main culprit that could lead to inadequate protein intake is the consumption of highly processed foodlike substances such as soda, candy, chips, and pretzels. These drinks and foods contain mostly carbohydrates and refined fats such as vegetable oils, and they're generally very low in protein.

All plants contain protein because they need it for proper structure and function. Animals ultimately get their protein (essential amino acids, to be precise) from plants, either by eating them directly or by eating other animals that eat plants. Still, plant protein differs from animal protein in many ways that have significant health implications, particularly for aging and life span.

The Difference Between Plant and Animal Protein

The simple word *protein* gives little away of its complexity. Carbohydrates are chains of sugar molecules, sometimes long and sometimes short. Fats (triglycerides) consist of three chains of fatty acids linked to a glycerol molecule. Proteins, however, can be of virtually any size and composition and contain different amounts and types of amino acids. They range from two amino acids linked together to chains that stretch hundreds of amino acids long.

Plants must synthesize all of their necessary amino acids, whereas animals eat plants to obtain the essential amino acids they cannot produce themselves. Except in very limited amounts, humans do not store protein or amino acids. Small amounts of amino acids exist in our bloodstreams at all times due to normal turnover of protein. Old tissues can be broken down into component amino acids, which can be recycled into newly built proteins. Cells are continually being degraded and rebuilt to rejuvenate tissues. Red blood cells, for example, survive for only about three months before being replaced. Nerve cells (neurons) often live for decades, which is why nerve injuries heal so slowly. Skin cells are replaced every few days.

Protein, either from diet or breakdown of tissue, is used for two main purposes:

- To build (or rebuild) tissues
- To be burned or stored as fuel (glycogen or body fat)

Because of the many different proteins in our bodies, we require specific types of amino acids in the right quantities. Because the body can't store amino acids, except in very limited amounts, we must eat the right amount and proportion of amino acids when we need them. This system seems precarious because nature does not email us a handy daily list of which proteins to eat. Anyway, most of the foods we want to eat (either animal or plant) might not be available at our convenience. During the turnover of proteins, most of the amino acid components can be recycled and used to build new proteins, so we don't have to obtain all of them through diet alone.

Some proteins are easier for us to use than others. This concept is known as the *biological value of proteins*, and it's expressed as a number from 0 to 100. A protein with a biological value of 100 contains all the amino acids in the right proportions for humans to use. Egg protein has a value of 100; gluten, the protein found in wheat, has a value of 64.

If you eat eggs, you can use 100 percent of its protein. If you eat wheat, you can use only 64 percent of its protein. Plant proteins generally have lower biological values than animal proteins because humans are biologically much closer to animals than plants. Plant proteins serve vastly different purposes than animal proteins, such as contributing to photosynthesis, and they have vastly different physiology. However, the generally lower protein content and biological value of plants do not necessarily mean that plant foods are not good sources of protein.

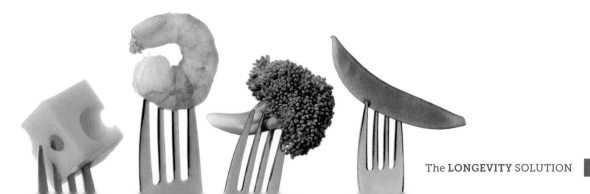

Protein Source	Bioavailability* Index
Whey protein isolate blends	100-159
Whey concentrate	104
Whole egg	100
Cow's milk	91
Egg white	88
Fish	83
Beef	80
Chicken	79
Casein	77
Rice	74
Wheat	64
Soy	59
Beans	49
Peanuts	43

*Bioavailability is the amount of protein that is absorbed in the body.

Vegans eat only plant foods and rarely experience severe protein deficiency. However, even minor deficiencies can cause health problems, and vegetables might not provide adequate amounts of all of the proteins necessary for humans. For example, lack of dietary niacin, also known as vitamin B3, may cause pellagra, which can present as delusions, diarrhea, inflamed mucous membranes, and scaly skin sores. This disease was previously quite widespread across the southern United States, where corn was a staple food to the exclusion of much else. The native tribes had traditionally treated corn kernels with an alkaline solution known as lime water, or they sometimes used wood ash. This treatment removed much of the aflatoxins (toxins found in the mold) and also increased the availability of the niacin in the corn. When people throughout the United States adopted corn as a staple crop, they didn't adopt the traditional preparation methods, which led to a pellagra epidemic. Lack of tryptophan, an amino acid, also can lead to pellagra because the body uses tryptophan to make niacin. In developed countries, pellagra is mostly a thing of the past.

Most animal proteins, like meat, eggs, milk, and cheese, are considered complete because they contain all nine essential amino acids. Most vegetables, by contrast, are not complete sources of protein. Eating a variety of vegetables is usually necessary to get all the essential proteins. The classic combination of rice and beans, for example, provides all the amino acids necessary for optimal health. Estimates suggest that people in the United States typically obtain about 70 percent of their protein from animal sources and 30 percent from plant sources.[2] Is this the optimal mix? A great way to get healthy sources of whole food plant protein is by eating organic nuts—such as almonds, hazelnuts, or cashews—from a company like Organic Traditions (http://organictraditions.com).

Animal Proteins

Animal and plant proteins differ mainly in their amino acid composition. Animal proteins contain more of the three branched-chain amino acids (BCAAs)—leucine, isoleucine, and valine—as well as the sulfur-containing amino acids cysteine and methionine.

Bodybuilders and other athletes often take BCAA supplements to increase muscle growth. They activate mechanistic target of rapamycin (mTOR), the cellular engine of growth and aging, and increase insulin-like growth factor 1 (IGF-1), which is great for building muscle. However, if longevity is your goal, this might not be so great because the enhanced growth might mean a shorter life. In the next few sections, we cover several different types of animal proteins, including their advantages and disadvantages.

 WHEY During cheese production, the curds are removed from the liquid milk portion, which contains proteins called *casein* and *whey*. Cow's milk contains approximately 20 percent whey protein, whereas human milk is about 60 percent whey protein. Whey contains a mixture of proteins, such as lactoglobulins and lactalbumin, which boost immunity and glutathione (an endogenous antioxidant). Whey also has displayed antiviral and antitumor effects.[3]

Undenatured whey has not been exposed to high heat and retains much of its original shape compared to the chemically processed whey often found in supplements. Studies in mice show that undenatured whey raises glutathione levels more than denatured whey[4] and that this effect may be protective against cancer.[5] Undenatured whey also enhances immune function.[6]

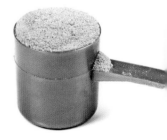

Protein Powder

Whey contains large amounts of the sulfur-containing amino acid cysteine, which is the critical rate-limiting factor in the production of glutathione, the body's most important internal antioxidant. Whey can potentially ameliorate oxidative stress and may be especially important for the elderly.

Ryse Supplements (https://rysesupps.com) makes a unique "loaded protein" that contains whey protein, MCTs, and organic prebiotic fiber. This supplement is particularly beneficial because it acts more like a whole food than an isolated protein.

Cysteine

Diabetics have low levels of glutathione and higher levels of oxidative stress. Cysteine supplementation (using the supplement N-acetylcysteine, or NAC) restored glutathione levels and reduced oxidative stress.[7]

NAC supplementation also might be useful for other conditions, including bipolar depression,[8] addiction, obsessive-compulsive disorders, and schizophrenia.[9] Human immunodeficiency virus (HIV) causes a massive loss of sulfur, which depletes glutathione.[10] Whey promotes weight gain and greater glutathione levels in HIV-positive individuals.[11]

Besides whey, the over-the-counter supplement NAC also supplies cysteine and thus replenishes glutathione. Cysteine itself is readily oxidized, which makes it difficult to store, but NAC does not oxidize, so it has a stable shelf life. During the metabolism of NAC, cysteine is liberated. NAC has a good safety profile, it's inexpensive, and there's even evidence that it can help people with chronic obstructive pulmonary disease (COPD) and influenza.[12]

Aging itself has been characterized as a "cysteine deficiency syndrome," and provision of cysteine in the form of whey or NAC can largely alleviate the oxidative stress and inflammation of aging.[13]

BCAAs

Whey is an especially rich source of easily digested BCAAs, mainly leucine, which makes it popular with bodybuilders, who often take about 20 grams of whey after exercise. The increased blood leucine level stimulates mTOR-favoring muscle growth more than other proteins, like casein or soy. This stimulation of mTOR might be useful in sarcopenia (muscle wasting) and cachexia (pathological loss of both lean and fat tissue, most often seen in cancer patients).[14] The high content of BCAAs in whey can overcome the anabolic resistance associated with aging. BCAAs also are used in treating liver cirrhosis.[15] In mice, supplementation with BCAAs might increase life span, perhaps due to increased mitochondrial activity and muscle mass.[16]

CASEIN

The other 80 percent of the protein in cow's milk is *casein* (Latin for "cheese"). In human milk, the percentage of casein varies from 20 to 45, depending on the stage of lactation. Until recently (in evolutionary terms), humans did not consume milk or milk products after weaning because lactose intolerance was almost universal in adults. Children have a lactose-metabolizing enzyme that would shut down after weaning. This changed about 5,000 years ago; this enzyme stayed active, so lactose tolerance began to spread. From that point, humans could drink milk from cows and other animals. Many people today, particularly from cultures that do not consume much dairy, are still lactose intolerant. Other people have allergies or intolerances (or both) to the proteins in cow's milk. However, there also are subtler problems.

Whereas whey can increase fasting insulin levels, casein stimulates the production of IGF-1,[17] which promotes muscle growth. However, overconsumption of casein may promote aging and cancer in animals,[18] although in humans, casein is not a carcinogen.

Cheese contains large amounts of casein but also plenty of healthy fats, vitamin K, and calcium. Most population studies find that eating high-fat dairy products is associated with weight loss, less diabetes, and lower death rates from heart disease and cancer. But, as with everything, balance is the key. Eating more than half a pound of cheese per day would likely accelerate aging and cancer. The dose makes the poison.

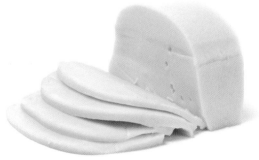

MEAT

Meat is the quintessential animal protein that humans have eaten for millions of years. However, the meat you buy from the supermarket today is not the same as the wild game your ancestors ate. The wild game had about seven times less total fat, three times less saturated fat, more omega-3, and less omega-6. Most primates are only occasional meat eaters, whereas humans vary widely from no meat to 100 percent meat. Some scientists believe that meat-eating was closely linked to the development of bigger brains. Archaeologists find that most large mammal species became extinct soon after the arrival of humans, suggesting that early humans preferentially hunted them for meat. Meat contains mainly protein and fat but little to no carbohydrate; the combination of protein and fat might have been necessary for enhanced brain growth.

Approximately 95 percent of Americans eat meat. The health effects of meat consumption are controversial, which is surprising, given our long history of meat-eating and its prevalence. Since the ascendancy of the cholesterol theory of heart disease in the late 1950s, we've been urged to eat less meat due to its high saturated fat and cholesterol content. But the truth isn't so simple. No large studies have ever found a link between eating saturated fat, cholesterol, or red meat and heart disease. The government has revised national dietary guidelines to state that dietary cholesterol presents no health problems.[19]

The purported link between meat and cancer, notably colon cancer, is controversial. The World Health Organization (WHO) recently declared that processed and red meats might cause cancer, though the effect is small. A daily portion of 2 ounces of processed meat or 3.5 ounces of red meat increases the risk of colon cancer from about 5 percent to 6 percent, according to the WHO.[20] If true, protein is probably not responsible for the increase because other meats (white meat) have as much or more protein. This association study cannot prove causation. Further, while the risk associated with red meat was marginal and controversial, it is hardly useful to lump processed meats with fresh meat, which has formed part of the human diet since humans came into existence.

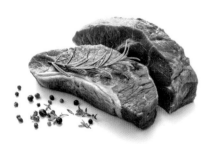

Consider fresh meat versus bologna. How are processed meats like bologna made? Well, you take the worst, most horrible cuts of meat (lungs, hooves, noses, and so on), grind them up so that you can't recognize all the yucky parts, and then shove in lots of sugar, chemicals, and seasonings, including MSG and other stuff, to cover all the terrible flavors. Then you shape it into something that looks vaguely like meat (sausages, sliced meats), package it nicely, and advertise the hell out of it. If you knew how they made hot dogs, you probably wouldn't eat them.

Ingredient lists on bologna often list "mechanically separated chicken or pork." What *is* that? Well, they take the chicken carcass and, after removing all the good meat, they fling the carcass around violently so that any remaining meat flies off the bone. Yes, all the eyeballs, nose hairs, lungs, and intestines are ground up into processed meat. This bologna, which looks appetizingly like sliced turkey or chicken, actually contains corn syrup, sodium lactate, sodium phosphates, autolyzed yeast, sodium dictate, sodium erythorbate (made from sugar), sodium nitrite, dextrose extractives, potassium phosphate, sugar, and potassium chloride. Here's what you need to know: Corn syrup is sugar. Dextrose extractives are sugar. Sugar is sugar. In other words, some form of sugar shows up three times in the ingredients list. Autolyzed yeast is MSG. It's all sugar and MSG to make things taste good. Aside from the sugar and MSG, this "meat" includes plenty of chemical preservatives, like nitrates and phosphates, too.

Does it seem reasonable to lump this unholy meat concoction together with grass-fed fresh beef? Hardly. And that's the point of one of our key messages: Eat real food. Don't eat processed carbohydrates. Just as importantly, don't eat processed meat or oil, either. Processed vegetable oils are not the same as natural fats (and we cover this in greater detail in Chapter 11).

Meat supplies a large amount of essential amino acids because it's higher in leucine and methionine than dairy and eggs. Steak and chicken have about double the leucine and methionine compared to eggs, whereas seafood has only about 50 percent more of these amino acids compared to eggs. Overconsumption of these two amino acids is implicated in aging. Eating more of the amino acid glycine, found in bone broth and collagen, may alleviate methionine toxicity.[21]

Animal protein in real foods also contains natural fats and other micronutrients like vitamin B12, the long-chain omega-3 fatty acids docosahexaenoic acid (DHA) and eicosapentaenoic acid (EPA) (especially in oceanic seafood and grass-fed or pastured meat), zinc, and iron. Iron can be a double-edged sword, though; it's good or bad for your health depending on whether you're malnourished or overnourished. People with iron deficiency anemia were traditionally advised to eat liver because it's a rich source of iron; however, people who have iron overload should avoid it.

BONE BROTH

The standard Western diet is low in the amino acid glycine, which may be responsible for helping to block the harmful cardio-metabolic effects of fructose.[22] Glycine mimics methionine restriction, which robustly extends the life span of lab animals. Glycine "pulls" methionine out of the biochemical cycle known as the trans-sulfuration pathway. For both of these reasons, adding glycine-rich foods to your diet is a healthy thing to do. One of the richest sources of glycine is bone broth, which is made by simmering bones for several hours. You can use the resulting broth as a base for soups, sauces, and many other recipes. Hydrolyzed collagen protein is also a great source of glycine, as one-third of the amino acids contained in collagen are glycine.

ANIMAL PROTEIN: TOO MUCH OR TOO LITTLE?

Because animal protein generally has a higher biological value than plant protein, most people view animal protein as being better for building muscle. This is true only if the focus is malnourishment, or too little protein, which for much of human history was a significant problem. But not today. Overnutrition is the major concern in the West, and this problem is metastasizing to the rest of the world. Currently, some 70 percent of the American population is overweight or obese, which has led to an epidemic of type 2 diabetes, which in turn increases the risk of other diseases, such as heart disease and cancer. Being overnourished is not the same as being well-nourished because eating highly processed junk food, which is mostly empty calories and is often the cause of being overnourished, does not prevent vitamin deficiencies. In a world where overnutrition is a primary concern, the higher biological value of animal protein may work against it. Paradoxically, animal protein may be *too* nutritious.

Plant Protein

Plant proteins are harder to digest than animal proteins, as evidenced by their lower biological value. However, plants can still provide a complete amino acid profile with fewer calories because plants have a lower fat content. Ground beef, for example, is 17 percent protein compared to 28 percent protein in lentils and 40 percent in tofu. Plant sources also contain healthy amounts of phytochemicals—popularly known as "antioxidants"—of which animal sources contain none. Phytochemicals, like sulforaphane in cruciferous vegetables (like broccoli and cabbage), can upregulate cancer defense mechanisms such as the Nrf2 system. Plant sources have more fiber, vitamin C, potassium, and magnesium, which are associated with lower blood pressure and lower risk of stroke and death.[23]

A novel finding of a recent large study of more than 170,000 people spanning several decades was that eating more plant protein was associated with a lower death rate.[24] Previous studies had focused on the total amount of protein rather than the source. Animal protein was associated with a higher death rate in only those people with other risk factors, such as smoking, being obese, or being sedentary. Further, only processed and red meats, not fish or poultry, were associated with the risk, and processed meat was the major offender. Substituting plant protein (and perhaps fish or poultry) for processed and red meats could perhaps reduce mortality.

VEGETARIANS AND VEGANS

Vegetarians avoid meat, but some eat eggs and dairy. Vegetarians are generally healthier and live longer than meat eaters, but this benefit may not be related to eating less meat; it could stem from other health-related lifestyle practices. Health-conscious people who do eat meat have death rates similar to the death rates of vegetarians.[25] General avoidance of processed and junk foods, more exercise, less smoking and alcohol, and lower body mass index explain most of the difference rather than eating less meat per se.

Vegans go even further than vegetarians, avoiding all animal products completely, including meat, eggs, and dairy. Plants are their sole protein source. To avoid protein deficiency, vegans must combine different types of plants to get the right balance of amino acids. A classic combination is rice and beans; the proteins in these two foods complement each other. Together, these proteins have a higher biological value than when you consume only one. Vegans also can lack other nutrients, such as vitamin B12, carnitine, zinc, vitamin K2, and iron.

Infants fed a vegan diet may develop protein deficiency,[26] so it is generally a bad idea to adopt this diet too early in life. Decreased growth rates may lead to shorter stature and delayed puberty.[27] For adults, who don't have any growth requirements, it is a different story because of the trade-off between growth and longevity. Vegan diets, low in essential amino acids, decrease the synthesis of the growth hormone pro-aging IGF-1. The amino acid methionine, a potent stimulus to IGF-1, tends to be low in plant proteins such as nuts and legumes. Certain IGF-1-dependent cancers, such as breast and colon cancer, occur less commonly in vegans.

When growth is important, as with children, eating more meat is beneficial. When longevity is more important, eating less meat might be beneficial. Perhaps this is why many children strongly prefer meat and animal proteins, and adults change their preference to vegetables over time. Dr. Fung has noticed this effect personally. As a child, he only ate vegetables when forced, but as he got older, he gravitated toward the salad bar and other vegetables.

LEGUMES

Legumes are seeds and include beans, chickpeas, lentils, and peas. They are a great source of plant protein and contain significant amounts of dietary fiber and polyphenols. For those who follow a vegetarian diet, legumes provide a significant portion of daily protein needs. Large-scale studies show that a diet high in beans may provide a small cardio-protective effect (4 to 9 percent) and perhaps a small weight loss effect as well.[28] A meta-analysis of twenty-one studies estimated that 1 cup of legumes per day reduced weight by 0.34 kilogram (0.75 pound), which is a small but potentially beneficial amount.

Beans and lentils are high in protein, and they contain healthy amounts of calcium and potassium. These foods might be particularly effective for weight loss because they provide enough protein to meet requirements and supply fiber, which creates a sense of fullness.

GO NUTS! Aside from eating more legumes and seeds, eating more nuts increases the potassium-containing, buffering bases that fight against an acidic bodily environment.[29] By emphasizing plant protein rather than animal protein, you can still meet your overall protein requirements, which is very important for the elderly and infirm, yet protect yourself against latent acidosis that's caused by the modern Western diet.

Nuts contain lots of protein, and they're a good plant source of healthy fats. Walnuts contain healthy omega-3 fats, which are seriously lacking in most Western diets. Almonds are high in fiber and calcium. Tree nuts (not peanuts) might protect against weight gain,[30] metabolic syndrome,[31] and heart disease.[32] People who eat nuts daily have about a 20 percent lower death rate than those who do not.[33] Studies on the health habits of Seventh-Day Adventists, who live around seven years longer than the average person, find that nut consumption is a huge factor; only non-smoking and low body mass index are more significant factors.[34] These results are only associations, but eating nuts in place of other foods, whether animal-derived or carbohydrate-dense, may very well offer protection against obesity and early death.

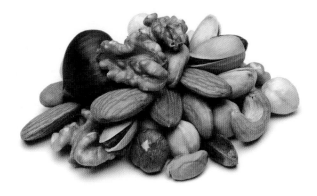

PROTEIN BARS

A great plant protein bar is IQ BAR (www.eatiqbar.com), which is a plant protein bar that comes in three flavors: Cacao Almond Sea Salt, Blueberry Lemon Sunflower, and Matcha Chai Hazelnut. The main ingredients include almonds, blueberries, sunflower seeds, and hazelnuts. IQ BARs are "real food" plant protein bars that provide 35 percent to 40 percent of the daily value for magnesium (a mineral that nearly 80 percent of the general population may be deficient in).

Advantages of IQ BAR (www.eatiqbar.com)

Plant protein

Ingredients that are real whole foods

Contains 35 to 40 percent of the daily value for magnesium

High in fiber

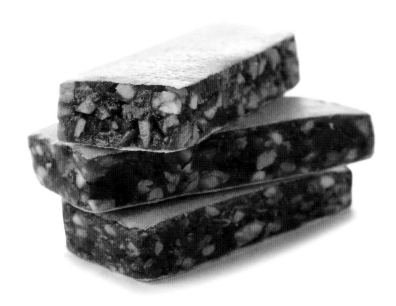

Comparing Plant and Animal Proteins

This section discusses the advantages and disadvantages of plant protein in comparison to animal protein. At the end of this section, we provide a summary table that compares the two types.

ANABOLIC RESPONSE

Different proteins provoke different anabolic (growth) responses. Consuming an adequate amount of protein is important for athletes and bodybuilders who are building strength but also for older people who need to maintain other lean tissues (including muscle and bone), which is robustly associated with good health.[35] If you are eating adequate protein, then the source makes little difference. Vegetarian and meat-containing diets were equally good at building muscle[36] when matched for total protein intake.[37]

Due to anabolic resistance, there is some data to suggest that in older people, eating only the recommended daily allowance (RDA) of protein (0.8 gram per kilogram per day) leads to muscle loss.[38] Taking more protein, whether plant or animal, can be useful. Plant protein doesn't have the excess leucine and methionine (which are pro-aging) that's in meat, but these two amino acids may help maximize muscle growth. You have to find a balance between growth and longevity.

Strength training supplemented by whey or pea protein can increase muscular growth. Pea protein contains amounts of leucine comparable to whey, but only half the methionine, which makes it a useful alternative.[39] Rice protein supplementation works, too, but you have to supplement with a fairly large amount (48 grams).[40]

HIGH-PROTEIN AND LOW-CARBOHYDRATE DIETS

A protein-rich diet that has a balance of plant and animal sources can lower blood pressure, improve lipid profiles, and reduce estimated cardiovascular risk.[41] From an evolutionary standpoint, our ancestors are estimated to have consumed about 50 percent protein from plants and 50 percent from animals.

High-protein diets, such as the Atkins diet, reduce refined carbohydrates and sugar, which is likely beneficial. A person who follows one of these diets may replace carbohydrates and sugar with more protein, but the protein is mostly from animal sources, and this substitution may not be optimal for health. Low-carbohydrate diets high in animal protein are associated with higher death rates from cardiovascular disease and cancer.[42] However, low-carbohydrate diets with more vegetable protein are associated with a lower death rate, particularly from cardiovascular disease.

The problem is not that meat is not nutritious. Instead, meat is too nutritious, which is not good in diseases of overnutrition and too much growth. Animal proteins stimulate more of the nutrient sensors insulin and mTOR than plant proteins do, and therefore animal proteins promote growth more. This effect is beneficial for malnourished people, which is why cavemen often hunted animals to extinction. But, in people suffering diseases of too much growth, the effect is not beneficial. In this situation, plant protein might be a better choice.

High-animal-protein diets may activate more IGF-1, which is implicated in the promotion of cancer. Lower levels of IGF-1 appear to protect centenarians against cancer—one reason they live that long.[43]

Eating less refined carbohydrates and sugar (less insulin), as well as targeted amounts of protein derived from animal sources (less mTOR), might be the best-case scenario. Eating less flour and sugar doesn't necessarily mean you must eat more meat and dairy. The Eco-Atkins diet encourages protein sources such as gluten, soy, nuts, vegetables, and grains, and it has been shown to improve lipid levels better than a low-fat diet that contains animal products.[44]

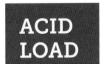

ACID LOAD

Animal protein is generally more acidic than plants, so our bodies must neutralize the acid load to avoid serious health implications, including osteoporosis, muscle loss (sarcopenia), kidney disease, and diabetes.[45] Ancestral diets are characterized by lots of animal protein, but they usually are balanced by equally large amounts of plant foods, which are often mildly alkaline.[46] Paleolithic (ancestral) diets are estimated to contain between 35 percent and 65 percent plants (by weight), which is close to our earlier estimate that humans likely evolved on a diet of approximately 50 percent animal and 50 percent plant foods, varying from season to season and geographic location. Even the Inuit in northern Canada consumed berries, seaweed, wild plants, and other plant material from the stomachs of their kill, thus maintaining long-term acid-base balance.

Modern diets generally contain less than half the amount of animal protein compared to ancestral diets and only about one-third the amount of natural plant foods. Instead, contemporary human diets are loaded with refined carbohydrates and sugars derived from grains but deficient in fiber, potassium, magnesium, and calcium. Certain grains—such as barley, oats, and quinoa—are mildly acidic or even alkaline, but, unfortunately, the most common grain we eat—wheat—is highly acidic.

Eating a typical Western diet with plenty of meat, grains, and sugar produces a lot of acid, which may deplete the body's buffering system. This depletion forces the body to rely on the minerals in bone and the amino acids, particularly glutamine (which is found in muscle), as a buffering system of last resort. Depletion can lead to osteoporosis and sarcopenia.

A study in women from thirty-three countries found that eating a lower ratio of vegetable to animal protein was associated with a significantly greater risk of hip fractures.[47] Germany had the highest risk for hip fracture incidence, followed by the Scandinavian countries, other European nations, and the United States. Countries such as China and Nigeria had a negligible rate of hip fractures.[48]

Osteoporosis often is believed to be caused by a lack of dietary calcium, but the evidence does not bear this out. Women in Japan and China eat less than one-third of the calcium of American women, but they have a much lower risk of osteoporosis. Neither is genetics a large factor. When Japanese women move to the United States, their risk of osteoporosis also moves up. Large-scale, randomized, controlled trials of calcium supplementation show no benefit in the reduction of fracture risk.[49]

The high-animal-protein Atkins diet increases net acid and calcium excretion. This result suggests that metabolic acidosis has increased and that bone might become calcium depleted.[50] Eating more plant proteins and fewer animal proteins may decrease the risk of osteoporosis and aging. Supplementation with bicarbonate or eating more fruits and vegetables to neutralize the acid is useful in select patient populations to improve mineral balance, bone resorption, bone formation, and kidney function.[51]

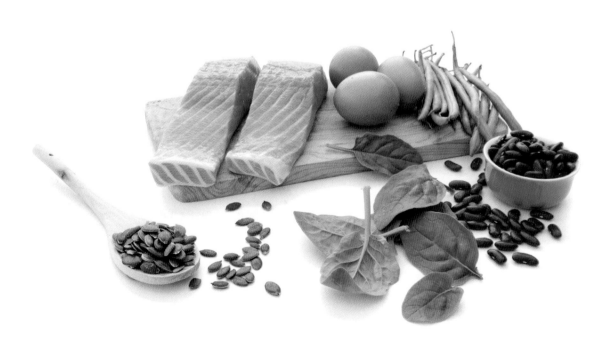

ANIMAL PROTEIN AND PLANT PROTEIN: A SIDE-BY-SIDE COMPARISON

	Animal Protein	Plant Protein
Advantages	Higher biological value, which means that the body can use it more effectively Provides certain vitamins (such as vitamins A, B12, D, and K2), minerals (zinc, sodium, and chloride), and other healthful constituents such as carnitine and choline (especially eggs) Greater activation of IGF-1 (pro-muscle, pro-growth, but also potentially pro-aging and pro-cancer)	Provides phytochemicals and fiber Provides greater amounts of certain vitamins and minerals (particularly copper, magnesium, and manganese) Provides alkalinity (improved bone health) Less bioavailable iron (decreased risk of iron overload)
Disadvantages	Acid load Iron overload Greater activation of IGF-1 (pro-growth, pro-aging, pro-cancer) Provides less of certain vitamins and minerals compared to plant protein (see Plant Protein Advantages)	Less activation of IGF-1 Fewer or lack of certain vitamins compared to animal protein (see Animal Protein Advantages) Might not be a complete source of essential amino acids

Recommendations

- Obtain about 50 percent of your daily protein needs from animal sources.
- Obtain about 50 percent of your daily protein needs from plant sources.
- Take your animal protein around periods of anabolic growth (such as childhood, pregnancy, and weightlifting).
- Elderly people, especially if sarcopenic, may need to consume greater amounts of protein.
- Consider supplementing with NAC and collagen and/or glycine.

06

THE OPTIMAL AMOUNT OF PROTEIN

Variation in the amount and type of protein consumed affects biological processes that are linked to health, aging, and disease. Finding the optimal amount of protein can yield big benefits, helping us to live longer and to experience fewer of the diseases and less of the frailty of aging. Too little protein causes disease. Too much protein causes disease. What's the right amount?

The Recommended Daily Allowance (RDA) set by the Institute of Medicine of the National Academy of Sciences to meet the minimal requirements of healthy adults is 0.8 gram per kilogram per day.[1] But the nitrogen balance method of determining protein requirements that they used is subject to large errors,[2] and some researchers believe the RDA has been significantly underestimated. They think the RDA should be 40 to 50 percent higher, at 1.2 grams per kilogram of body weight as a safe population-wide recommendation. (That's 84 grams of protein per day for an adult who weighs 70 kilograms [154 pounds].)

The RDA is only an average, and protein requirements vary greatly depending on whether a person is a child, an adult, elderly, pregnant, an athlete, in ill health or frail, obese, or is losing or gaining weight (or desiring to do so). The official dietary recommendations are intended to prevent deficiency rather than to suggest optimal protein intake for longevity, which is understandable given that knowledge of how protein affects longevity is relatively new.

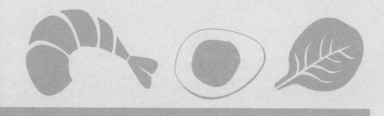

Our food is composed of three main macronutrients: fats, carbohydrates, and protein. Fats and carbohydrates are chiefly sources of energy, although there are a small number of essential fatty acids, whereas there is no such thing as an essential carbohydrate. Protein is different. Its primary function is for growth and maintenance rather than providing energy. Thus, the chief difference in protein requirements reflects the need for growth. In adults, there is little need for growth, except if you are trying to build muscle. An adult's liver, lungs, and kidney do not need to get any larger. In an infant, though, all organs and muscles need to grow, which means that an infant has a much higher protein requirement for its body weight. The infant must grow from less than 10 pounds to more than 100 pounds, and that growth requires more protein. Also, a person who has a higher lean mass—the entire body excluding fat tissue and water—has a higher protein requirement. However, there is an upper limit of protein use. You can't gain muscle only by eating lots of protein; otherwise, we'd all look like bodybuilders just from eating more protein.

Severe protein deficiency is rare in developed countries, but the amount that prevents deficiency and the optimal amount are not the same. If a person consumes less than the minimal amount of protein, loss of lean mass (especially muscle) and decreased antioxidant capacity could result.[3] Whereas most people in the Western world already consume this higher amount of protein (about 70 percent coming from animal sources and 30 percent coming from plant sources[4]), some do not, notably among the elderly. In hospitals, older people with protein malnutrition are often admitted; they're referred to as "tea and toasters." These frail, elderly people had difficulty cooking, so they would eat mostly tea and toast, which contain very little protein.

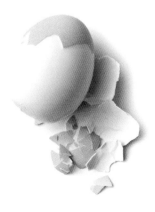

Protein for Growth and Development

People in a life stage when growth and development is a priority, such as pregnant women, infants, children, and adolescents, should eat more protein. Estimated protein requirements vary with the rate of growth of infants over the first year of life, ranging from an estimated 2 grams per kilogram of body weight at the age of one to two months to about 1.3 grams per kilogram at six months of age and then to about 1.0 gram per kilogram at one year.[5] The protein content of human milk, as well as its ratio of casein to whey proteins, changes during that time; evolution has optimized milk to suit the infant's needs. The American Academy of Pediatrics recommends exclusive breastfeeding for the first six months of life; after that time, breastfeeding may continue as the child begins to eat other foods, to one year or longer.[6]

As a child ages, the protein requirement slowly declines; by ten years of age, a safe level of protein is about 0.9 gram per kilogram, which is a level only slightly higher than for an adult. In early pregnancy, a woman's protein requirement is estimated to be about 1.2 grams per kilogram; in late pregnancy, her requirement is about 1.5 grams.[7]

Protein for the Elderly

Protein requirements for the elderly are different than for other adults. They have *increased* protein needs because they cannot use protein with the same efficiency as younger adults. Failure to meet those increased needs can result in loss of muscle and other lean mass, lower antioxidant capacity, and lower immune function, all of which play a role in increased risks of illness and frailty.

Losing skeletal muscle (sarcopenia) with age affects health in many ways. Muscle acts as a "metabolic sink" by taking up nutrients and contributing to overall insulin sensitivity. Sarcopenia is a major cause of falls and bone fractures, and it can leave an elderly person unable to perform normal activities of daily living, such as getting out of a chair unassisted, which may lead to placement in a nursing home.

Sarcopenia is most commonly due to lack of activity. The adage "use it or lose it" is applicable. Prolonged bed rest, such as during hospitalization or major illness, results in a large loss of muscle mass. One study of healthy elderly patients found an astounding loss of 1 kilogram of muscle even while subjects were consuming adequate protein.[8] Sedentary behavior, although not as extreme as bed rest, also contributes to sarcopenia. For this reason, strength training, especially when combined with extra or different types of protein, can be a boon for the elderly.

Also, anabolic resistance contributes to sarcopenia. Skeletal muscle undergoes a normal cycle of turnover—muscle breakdown balanced by protein synthesis. Anabolic resistance increases with age, and muscle protein synthesis in response to dietary protein decreases; the result is a decline in muscle mass. Lack of exercise, inflammation, and oxidative stress also can contribute to anabolic resistance.

Increased dietary protein can overcome anabolic resistance to help maintain muscle.[9] A consensus statement from a group of experts, the PROT-AGE Study Group, made the following statements and recommendations:

- To maintain and regrow muscle, older people require more protein than younger people; older people should consume an average of 1.0 to 1.2 grams per kilogram of body weight daily.

- The amount of protein at one meal that increases muscle growth (i.e., that overcomes anabolic resistance) is higher in older people, at about 25 to 30 grams of protein per meal, equivalent to about 2.5 to 2.8 grams of leucine per meal.

- When possible, older individuals should perform endurance exercise 30 minutes a day and resistance exercise (strength training) 10 to 15 minutes or more, two or three times per week, if it is safe and tolerable for the individual.

- Protein supplementation, such as a whey drink, especially before or right after exercise, might help older people regain muscle. Whey has been shown to be more effective for muscle growth than casein. Bodybuilders are well known to ingest protein immediately before or after strength training to increase muscle growth, and exercise physiologists have studied this practice extensively. It works.

- Most older people with an acute or chronic disease (except kidney disease) need even more protein, in the range of 1.2 to 1.5 grams per kilogram of body weight daily.

- Older people with severe illness or injury or who have marked malnutrition might need as much as 2.0 grams per kilogram of body weight daily.

Eating one high-protein meal (known as "protein pulse feeding") is more effective than distributing the protein equally over the day. Omega-3 fatty acid supplementation also augments the increase in muscle growth caused by dietary protein; regular supplementation with fish oil or other supplements that contain omega-3 fatty acids can help older people retain and regain muscle.[10]

Hospitalization, which sometimes involves forced immobility, often results in weight loss, particularly in undernourished patients. An estimated 40 percent of hospital patients are malnourished, as defined by a body mass index of less than 20.[11] This malnourishment puts them at risk of infections, and hospital-acquired infections are an increasing problem. The CDC estimated that in 2011, more than 720,000 cases of hospital-acquired infection occurred, which is about 1 in 25 people.[12]

Extra dietary protein can help this situation. In a geriatric population, provision of 8 grams a day of essential amino acids cut the infection rate by about 30 percent, while also increasing hemoglobin and improving other health markers.[13] Trauma patients who received a formula containing whey protein also had a much lower incidence of infections.[14] As for muscle, providing essential amino acids ameliorates muscle loss during bed rest.[15]

Protein for Athletes

Building muscle requires protein[16] but also salt. During metabolism, stomach acid (hydrochloric acid) and pepsin break down dietary protein into peptide fragments and free amino acids. The amino acids pass into the small intestine, where absorption occurs. Antacids and medications that block stomach acid, such as commonly prescribed proton pump inhibitors, prevent normal digestion of proteins. Low-salt diets also reduce stomach acid by reducing the availability of chloride. Eating too many refined foods, especially with reduced stomach acid, might also lead to overgrowth of bacteria in the small intestine, known as small intestinal bacterial overgrowth (SIBO), which might impair protein absorption.

Low-salt diets also promote muscle insulin resistance, which can reduce muscle growth and cause overtraining syndrome (exercising in excess of the body's ability to recover), muscle cramps, and muscle spasms that reduce your ability to exercise.[17]

> You need to muscle-up by salting-up, especially before exercise. Dr. DiNicolantonio's previous book, *The Salt Fix,* provides the precise salt intake dosing that you should use before exercise.

After the intestine has absorbed amino acids, the gut and liver use approximately half the amino acids. Known as "first pass" clearance, this means about 50 percent of the protein you consume isn't even available for muscle growth. Importantly, branched-chain amino acids (BCAAs) are metabolized less by the liver, so they may be especially beneficial for muscle growth because of increased availability.[18]

Once the amino acids hit your systemic circulation, only about 10 percent goes toward skeletal muscle protein synthesis. The rest is used for energy (gluconeogenesis) or as building blocks for proteins and neurotransmitters throughout the body.[19] Muscle protein synthesis begins about 30 minutes after amino acid absorption and peaks at around 2 hours. Increased blood amino acids stimulate muscle growth, but only up to a certain point.

Maximum muscle protein synthesis occurs with a protein intake of 0.24 gram per kilogram of body mass per meal in younger males (generally 50 years old or younger) and 0.40 gram per kilogram in older adults due to anabolic resistance.[20] Muscle protein synthesis varies depending on the type and intensity of exercise. If you're trying to build muscle, then eating 20 grams of protein every three hours might be appropriate for you because that schedule optimizes muscle protein synthesis throughout the day. A general rule is that young men generally can get maximal protein synthesis per meal if they consume 20 to 30 grams of protein; older adults need around 40 grams.[21]

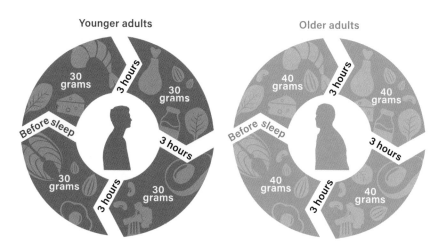

Fig. 6.1: The 30 rule and the 40 rule

Eating more protein (40 grams versus 20 grams) can stimulate more muscle growth, but the benefits are marginal.[22] Indeed, most athletes can satisfy their protein requirements by consuming around 30 grams of protein at each meal (0.24 to 0.30 gram per kilogram). However, pre-sleep doses of protein may need to be higher than 30 grams to maximize overnight skeletal muscle anabolism.[23] To summarize, younger adults use the "30 rule": consume 30 grams of protein per meal at least 3 hours apart and 30 grams of protein before going to sleep. Older adults should use the "40 rule": consume 40 grams of protein per meal 3 hours apart and 40 grams of protein before going to sleep. Most adults should have an overall daily protein intake between 1.6 and 2.2 grams per kilogram for optimizing muscle mass growth with resistance exercise.[24] A good general rule prescribes *1 gram of protein for every 1 pound of body weight* (equal to 2.2 grams of protein per kilogram).

Athletes need about double the amount of protein for optimal performance (1.6 to 1.8 grams per kilogram per day) that sedentary people need (0.8 gram per kilogram per day).[25] However, the amount varies widely depending on many interacting factors, like energy and carbohydrate intake; type, intensity, and duration of exercise; dietary protein quality; training history; gender; age; and timing of protein consumption. One size does not fit all. Lean athletes who are resistance-trained may need upward of 3 grams per kilogram per day of protein to prevent muscle losses during energy restriction.[26]

Athletes often are encouraged to drink sugary sports drinks. Glucose stimulates insulin secretion, which encourages muscle growth. However, this requires only around 5 IU/mL of insulin; higher doses do not enhance this effect.[27] In other words, you don't need sugar to build muscle. Most normal diets have sugar levels many times higher than what is needed.

Athletes should consume glycine as a supplement powder or capsule or as hydrolyzed collagen protein in addition to consuming protein from traditional sources. The body needs around 15 grams of glycine per day to meet both collagen and noncollagen synthesis requirements. However, the typical American diet provides only around 1.5 to 3 grams of glycine per day. The body can synthesize small amounts of glycine (around 3 grams per day), but the shortfall is still approximately 10 grams of glycine daily for almost everyone.[28] Dr. DiNicolantonio's research has shown that glycine taken at doses of 5 grams three times a day can benefit those with metabolic syndrome by reducing oxidative stress and systolic blood pressure.[29]

PRACTICAL RECOMMENDATIONS FOR HIGH-PERFORMANCE ATHLETES

- Aim to eat approximately 0.4 gram per kilogram of body mass of protein per meal.

- Space protein-containing meals three to five hours apart.

- Ingest around 30 to 40 grams of protein one to three hours before going to sleep to offset the effects of the overnight fast.

- When you're performing resistance exercise, eat 1.6 to 2.2 grams of protein per kilogram per day distributed among three to four meals.

- Consider taking glycine supplements.[30]

RECOMMENDATIONS FOR ATHLETES IN ENERGY RESTRICTION

- Because daily protein requirements are greater for preserving lean body mass, consume around 2.3 to 3.1 grams per kilogram per day of protein. Those who are more overweight and exercise-naive should aim for the lower end of this range, whereas leaner resistance-trained individuals should aim for the higher end of this range.

- Perform resistance exercise during energy restriction to preserve lean body mass.

- Ensuring adequate protein intake helps appetite control during energy restriction.[31]

ENDURANCE ATHLETES

It would seem obvious that bodybuilders require more protein than other people. But oddly enough, they require only 1.05 grams of protein per kilogram of body weight (around 73.5 grams of protein per day for a 70-kilogram [154-pound] bodybuilder), which is only about 10 percent more than sedentary people require. Endurance athletes require far more protein; they need about 70 percent more (about 1.37 grams of protein per kilogram per day) than sedentary people. Less intensive endurance training may only require 0.97 gram of protein per kilogram per day. A safe level would be 1.6 grams of protein per kilogram per day for endurance athletes and 1.2 grams of protein per kilogram per day for bodybuilders.[32] (See the "Protein Recommendations for Health and Activity Conditions" table at the end of the chapter for more specifics.) Bodybuilders often supplement with protein, but runners and other endurance athletes often do not, which puts them at risk of deficiency.

It's important to note that these safe margins of intake are based on a diet that is approximately 50 percent carbohydrate. Increased workout intensity or a lower carbohydrate intake may necessitate higher levels of protein. Additionally, pregnant and lactating women and adolescent athletes likely require more protein.[33]

Overtraining—which is characterized by fatigue, infections, and poor athletic performance—often sets in for elite and Olympic-level athletes, and it might be due partially to inadequate protein intake.[34] Researchers found that when fatigued athletes consumed an extra 20 to 30 grams of protein a day, blood amino acid patterns returned to normal, and many of them overcame their fatigue to resume regular training at their previous level.

To summarize:

- Protein requirements for athletes depend on many factors.
- Strength athletes need only a little more protein than sedentary people.
- Endurance athletes need much more protein than sedentary people (at least 1.6 grams of protein per kilogram per day).
- Inadequate protein intake during intense training may lead to overtraining syndrome.

Protein for Weight Loss

When people lose weight, the lost weight isn't entirely body fat; some of it is muscle. Although overweight and obese people tend to carry more muscle than people of normal weight, in general, we want to avoid losing muscle. Muscle mass and strength correlates with health and long life.[35] As much as 25 percent of the weight lost using low-calorie diets is muscle,[36] which can sometimes be mitigated by eating more protein.[37]

Adding resistance exercise and more protein to a low-calorie diet not only can abolish muscle loss but actually can help you add muscle as you lose fat. Whey protein has been well studied, but casein supplements might be more effective, with some studies showing more fat loss, more lean mass gain, and a greater increase in strength with casein.[38] Whey is a fast-digesting protein, whereas casein is a slow-digesting protein; therefore, each protein supplement has unique advantages. Whey causes a spike in plasma amino acids that are useful for athletes immediately after training. Casein taken just before bedtime slowly releases amino acids, which prevents muscle breakdown and promotes muscle protein synthesis throughout the night.

Higher protein intake is often useful in weight loss because of its satiating effect. Eating protein increases satiety hormones like peptide YY. Think about eating a small piece of steak or chicken in comparison to drinking an equal-calorie portion of soda. You can drink the soda without feeling the slightest bit fuller than when you started, but the steak or chicken will make you feel full and keep you feeling full for longer. This feeling of satiety is beneficial in weight-loss efforts. Protein's role in obesity has been a relatively neglected area of study because protein typically makes up only about 15 percent of food energy, and protein consumption has remained nearly the same throughout the obesity epidemic.

The *protein leverage hypothesis* of obesity suggests that eating food relatively dilute in protein leads to obesity.[39] Eating foods low in protein may result in an innate physiological drive to eat more food overall to get adequate protein, which leads to weight gain. Junk foods like chips and soda are low in protein. Official dietary recommendations to eat a low-fat diet coincided with the start of the obesity epidemic. Eating low-fat foods also might have led to eating low-protein foods because many foods that are high in fat, such as meat, are also high in protein.

The Optimal Amount of Protein

Optimal protein intake varies depending on goals and underlying health conditions. People who are older, ill, or immobilized need more protein to maintain good muscle tone and health. Athletes need more protein than nonathletes, but not nearly as much as common lore suggests.

Consuming more protein can reduce hunger and increase muscle growth. Although protein restriction doesn't make much sense for those who exercise on a regular basis, consuming too much protein may also have some negative consequences.

PROTEIN RECOMMENDATIONS FOR HEALTH AND ACTIVITY CONDITIONS[40]

Population	Recommended Amount of Protein Daily (g/kg body weight)	Recommended Types of Protein	Notes
Adults who engage in moderate exercise	1.2–1.8 g/kg, the RDA	A mix of animal and plant proteins	Low to moderate exercise—e.g., walking—does not demand extra protein.
Endurance athletes	1.6–1.8 g/kg	Emphasis on animal proteins with high BCAA	Moderate to high-intensity exercise for relatively long durations—e.g., running or cycling.
Bodybuilders and strength athletes	1.6–3.3 g/kg	Emphasis on animal proteins with high BCAA	After initial training, bodybuilding requires less protein than commonly assumed.
Elite athletes	1.7–3.3 g/kg	Emphasis on animal proteins; amino acid supplementation might be appropriate	Highly competitive athletics—e.g., collegiate, professional, Olympic athletic competition.
Elderly and sedentary people	1.2 g/kg	A mix of animal and plant proteins	More protein necessary to maintain and build muscle and bone.
Kidney disease patients (glomerular filtration rate < 25 ml/min) not undergoing dialysis	0.6 g/kg	Emphasis on plant proteins	Less protein may inhibit disease progression.[41]
Kidney disease patients undergoing dialysis	1.2 g/kg	A mix of animal and plant protein	Higher protein needed to prevent muscle wasting.[42]
Hospitalized or bedridden patients	25–30 g with each meal	Emphasis on high-quality proteins with BCAA	Prevents muscle loss and prevents infections via better immunity.[43]

Maximal stimulation of muscle protein synthesis may require at least 0.24 gram of protein per kilogram per meal for younger adults (20 to 29 years old) and 0.40 gram per kilogram for older adults (older than 50).

PROTEIN RECOMMENDATIONS BASED ON TYPE OF WORKOUT

Training Type	Protein Recommendation	Recommended Protein Type	Notes
Strength training, bodybuilding, pre-workout	25 g; more, up to 40 g, might be better for those with higher body weight (>150 lbs.), who are older, or who are doing whole body or large muscle group workouts[44]	Whey protein	Take protein before workout or after workout within two hours.
Running, endurance training	25 g post-training	Whey protein	Post-training is likely better than pre-training.
Gymnastics, wrestling, swimming, football, and so on	25 to 40 g post-training	Whey or casein protein	Whey is digested quickly; casein is slow.
Low- to moderate-intensity exercise	Normal protein meal	All types	Extra protein isn't required.

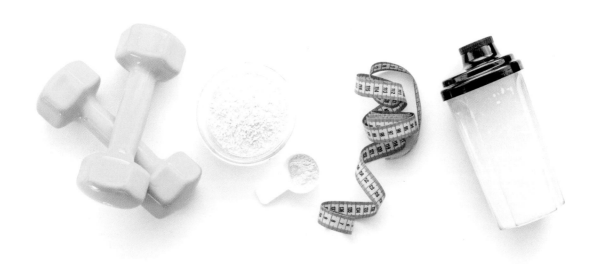

07
FASTING

Fasting, the voluntary abstinence from eating food, has been used throughout human history for various purposes, including religious, health, and spiritual. Whether you call it a *fast*, a *cleanse*, or *detoxification*, the idea is that periodic restriction of all foods is a healthy habit. In fact, all major religions embrace fasting as a cornerstone of healthy living.

Fasting is one of the keys to longevity because it improves all the dietary factors we've talked about so far. It restricts calories and protein. It reduces insulin and mTOR and activates AMPK and autophagy. These benefits are delivered at no cost and without taking any time. Fasting is not something you do; it's something you do NOT do. It can both simplify and enrich your life. So why has this ancient tradition been largely abandoned? People practiced fasting for millennia, but it has been only recently that many people have started to believe that fasting is harmful because it may cause malnutrition as the body metabolizes its own protein for energy.

You should not confuse malnutrition from not eating, which is called *wasting*, with fasting. Wasting is a pathological situation in which the body has inadequate stores of body fat and is therefore forced to burn functional tissue such as muscle to provide the energy needed to survive. Metabolism of muscle for energy can cause weakness and, in extreme situations, death. These severe outcomes typically happen when a person has a body fat percentage lower than 4 percent. By contrast, a typical American male carries 25 to 30 percent body fat and females carry 35 to 40 percent body fat, although this varies by age. Even an elite marathon runner, who might not have any obvious visible fat, still carries approximately 10 percent body fat.

We can use a quick calculation to see at what point the body is in danger of wasting. A man who weighs 180 pounds and stands 5 feet 11 inches has a body mass index of 25 (normal). With average body fat of 25 percent, he carries 45 pounds of body fat (180 lbs x 0.25 = 45 pounds of body fat). A pound of fat supplies approximately 3,500 calories of energy—enough for two days. With 45 pounds of body fat, this man carries enough body fat to sustain him for ninety days, or almost three months straight, without eating any food whatsoever before he is in danger of wasting. As we discuss in more detail later, during extended periods without food, the body burns mostly fat, with some protein breakdown. In general, as long as an individual's micronutrient intake is adequate, the loss of protein (much of it coming from the skin and damaged proteins) does not appear to be life-threatening—even when it continues for months.

The three-month estimate is an underestimate because the body's basal metabolism, or the rate of consumption of energy, will fall as the person loses weight. An obese or overweight person can survive even longer before wasting is a real concern. By contrast, most people are concerned if they go more than three hours between breakfast and lunch without eating.

Fasting should also not be confused with starvation, which is an involuntary condition. There's a stark contrast between starvation and fasting. During starvation, no food is available, regardless of whether the person wants to eat. Fasting is a fully conscious decision to abstain from food, even though food is readily available. The photos of children without adequate nutrition in Africa show starvation. These children do not eat because no food is available; going without eating is not a choice for them. Because fasting is an entirely voluntary process, a person may stop fasting at any point.

The possibilities for fasting are infinite. We offer some suggestions in Chapter 13, but if you're looking for a more detailed plan for starting a fasting regimen, Dr. Fung's book *The Complete Guide to Fasting* is a great resource.

Furthermore, when fasting for health reasons, remember that you should not start a fasting regimen unless your medical doctor is closely monitoring your health status and states that you are healthy enough to fast. And if you do not feel well for any reason at any time during your fast, you should stop immediately and seek help from an experienced practitioner.

Fears about fasting are highly prevalent. We constantly hear that we must eat, eat, and eat—even when we want to lose weight! If neither malnutrition nor being underweight is a concern, the fear of "burning muscle" (which mostly comes from nitrogen balance studies) during periods of fasting has not been backed up by practical experience, the known physiology of fasting, or clinical studies. (Nitrogen loss does not necessarily mean muscle loss; it can be due to the loss of excess skin and damaged proteins that comes with fasting.)

Let's examine the physiology of fasting and what happens to protein metabolism when you fast.

The Physiology of Fasting

During fasting, the body must rely upon its stores of food energy for basal metabolic needs. Although we mostly think about the body's energy expenditure in terms of exercise, our body requires a significant amount of energy to keep our vital organs (the brain, heart, lungs, and kidneys) running properly. All that functionality is largely controlled unconsciously by our autonomic nervous system. Even when we're bed-bound, our bodies still need energy to keep this machinery going. If we eat nothing (fasting), there is no incoming food energy, and we must rely completely on our stored food energy to survive.

HOW DOES THE BODY STORE FOOD ENERGY?

The body stores food energy in two main ways.

- Glycogen in the liver

- Body fat

When we eat, the level of the hormone insulin goes up and instructs our body to store some of the incoming food energy. Glucose from carbohydrates is strung together into long chains called *glycogen*, which is stored in the liver. When we eat protein, we break down and absorb the component amino acids. These are used to build any necessary new proteins. However, if we eat more than we need, the body has no way of storing excess amino acids.

Fig. 7.1: Differences between a fed state and a fasted state on the body's use of food energy

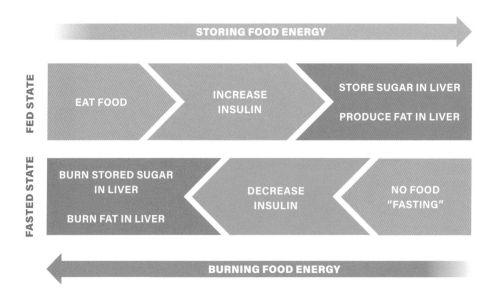

Fed versus fasted state: storing versus burning energy

Instead, the body turns those excess proteins into glucose to store that food energy. The average American who eats a standard diet is estimated to turn 50 to 70 percent of the protein they ingest into new glucose molecules.[1] In other words, the average diet exceeds the protein needs of the body by a fairly large margin.

Glycogen is a useful storage form of energy, but the liver has limited storage space. Once glycogen has maxed out, the body converts the excess glucose into triglycerides, or fat, by a process known as *de novo lipogenesis*. These newly created fat molecules can then be exported out of the liver and into the fat cells for long-term storage.

The two storage systems are complementary. The glycogen system is simple but limited in storage capacity. The body fat system is much more complex and requires the body to change molecules of carbohydrates and proteins to fat (triglycerides). However, the advantage is that the body fat system is almost limitless in its capacity.

The two systems are analogous to the way we use a refrigerator (the glycogen system) and a freezer (the body fat system). We store excess food in two different ways. We can store food in the refrigerator and both putting food in and taking it out are easy. However, a refrigerator has limited capacity. When the refrigerator is full, we can freeze the food. Storing food in a freezer is more difficult because we must package it properly and freeze it; however, we have unlimited storage because we can always add another freezer in the basement of our house.

WHAT HAPPENS DURING FASTING?

During fasting, the food energy storage process reverses. Insulin falls, and that decline is the signal that the body should start using some of the stored food energy to power the body. Dr. George Cahill described the five stages between eating and prolonged starvation/fasting. (Four stages are shown in Figure 7.2.[2]) In the first four hours after you have eaten, insulin is high, and you are still mostly drawing from the glucose you have eaten. All the tissues of the body can use this glucose, and you are still storing food energy as glycogen. Once the glycogen store is full, any excess must be turned into body fat.

By stage 2 (four to sixteen hours after eating), the exogenous glucose is no longer available as a source of energy, so you must rely on body stores. The most readily available source of energy is glycogen in the liver. You break down the glycogen into its component glucose molecules and send it out to the body for energy. Those glycogen stores last approximately twenty-four hours. So, if you are not exercising, even up to twenty-four hours of fasting does not necessarily force the body to burn either fat or protein.

By stage 3 (sixteen to thirty hours after eating), the stores of glycogen are starting to run out. Body fat is not yet available, so you bridge the gap by producing glucose from protein in a process called *gluconeogenesis*, which means "the creation of new glucose." During this stage, your body transitions from using glucose, which is increasingly becoming scarce, to using fat and protein, which is becoming available from body stores. This area is what concerns many people because they believe that this breakdown of protein constitutes muscle loss. These concerns are largely misplaced for reasons we discuss in more detail later in this chapter.

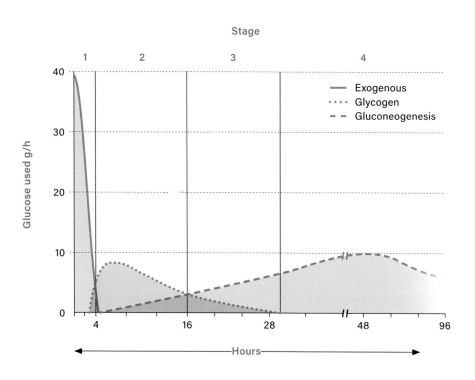

Stage	1	2	3	4
Origin of blood glucose	Exogenous	Glycogen Hepatic gluconeogenesis	Hepatic gluconeogenesis Glycogen	Gluconeogenesis, hepatic and renal
Tissues using glucose	All	All except liver, muscle, and adipose tissue of diminished rates	All except liver, muscle, and adipose tissue of rates intermediate between stages 2 and 4	Brain, RBCS, renal medulla, small amount by muscle

Most of our organs and muscles can use fat (triglycerides) directly. The brain, however, cannot use fat directly because of the blood-brain barrier. Also, because the brain requires so much energy, it would quickly deplete the available glucose. The liver compensates by producing ketone bodies from the body fat. These ketones can cross the blood-brain barrier so the brain can use them as an energy source. An estimated 60 to 75 percent of the brain's energy can be derived from ketones, which significantly reduces the need for glucose because much of it must be produced from protein.

During stage 4 (thirty hours to twenty-four days after eating), the body mobilizes stores of body fat for energy. By this point, most tissues of the body have switched to burning triglycerides for energy. Only the brain, the red blood cells, and the inner part of the kidney must still use glucose. Some of the glycerol backbone of the triglyceride molecule is turned into glucose, and a small amount is still derived from the breakdown of protein. The only substantial difference is that the amount of protein breakdown is further reduced. During extended fasting, the body mostly burns fat.[3] This is logical because the body mostly stores food energy as fat.

This entire process of extended fasting essentially describes the shift in energy metabolism from glucose (from food and glycogen) to body fat. Although there is still some breakdown of protein, as we discuss later in this chapter in the section "Glucose Requirements and Protein Breakdown," the clinical studies show that with twenty-four hours of fasting the body does not increase the "burning" of protein for energy. Indeed, long-term studies indicate that the body doesn't ramp up protein metabolism. However, because of the continued oxidation of protein, some people are apprehensive that this could result in muscle or organ wasting. Should you be concerned?

Clinical Studies

Involuntary periodic starvation or its voluntary counterpart (fasting) has been part of human nature since the beginning of time. Until relatively recently, food was not always available. To survive the hard times, early humans needed to store food energy as body fat when food was abundant. If humans did not have an efficient storage and retrieval method of food energy, our species would have died long ago.

After food availability became more reliable, most human cultures and religions prescribed voluntary periods of fasting. For example, Jesus was said to have fasted for forty days and forty nights, and many subsequent followers have undertaken this themselves without significant health damage. Many Muslims fast during the holy month of Ramadan, and also regularly twice a week during the rest of the year. In these situations, fasting was considered a cleansing procedure without any connotation of harmful muscle burning.

The repeated feeding-fasting cycles inherent in prehistory times did not seem to have any detrimental effect on muscle mass. Descriptions of traditional societies such as the Native Americans or Inuit of North America or tribesmen in Africa suggest they were lively and energetic rather than emaciated and weak. Descriptions of modern followers of the Greek Orthodox Church, with its many days of fasting, do not include portrayals of lethargy and weakness. It is virtually impossible that humans, who were designed to store food energy as body fat, would burn muscle when food was not available. If they did, all people throughout history until the twentieth century who followed this feast-famine cycle either through periodic starvation or fasting would be almost pure fat. Instead, they were lean and strong.

Recent clinical evidence bears out the fact that alternating twenty-four-hour periods of repeated fasting/feeding does not cause muscle loss. In a 2010 study of alternate-day fasting, patients were able to lose significant fat mass with no change in lean mass. In this schedule, subjects eat on a normal schedule on feeding days; on the alternate days, they fast. Also, the researchers noted numerous metabolic benefits—such as reduced cholesterol, triglycerides, and waist circumference—along with the weight loss.[4]

A more recent 2016 study compares a strategy of intermittent fasting with daily calorie restriction (the conventional method of weight loss suggested by most health professionals).[5] Both groups lost a comparable amount of weight, but the intermittent fasting group lost only 1.2 kilogram of lean mass compared to 1.6 kilograms in the calorie restriction group. When we compare the percentage increase in lean mass, we see that the fasting group *increased* by 2.2 percent compared to 0.5 percent in the calorie restriction group, implying that fasting may be up to four times better at preserving lean mass according to this measure. Importantly, the fasting group lost more than double the amount of the more dangerous visceral fat.

The same study highlighted some other important benefits, too. Chronic calorie restriction reduced basal metabolic rate, where intermittent fasting did not. Because fasting (but not chronic calorie restriction) induces the counter-regulatory hormones, the body is switching fuel sources, rather than shutting itself down. Further, chronic calorie restriction increases ghrelin, the hunger hormone, where fasting did not. If you are less hungry with fasting compared to calorie restriction, you are more likely to stick to the diet. Both of these are overwhelming advantages for weight loss.

Despite the concerns that fasting may cause loss of muscle, our long human experience and multiple human clinical trials show the exact opposite. Intermittent fasting preserves lean tissue better than conventional weight-loss methods. Thinking again about gluconeogenesis, at first glance, this seems counterintuitive. If intermittent fasting causes gluconeogenesis (turning protein into glucose), how can it possibly be better at preserving muscle? Part of the answer lies in the fact that gluconeogenesis does not start until approximately 24 hours after the last meal. The other part of the answer lies in the hormonal adaptation to fasting—the counter-regulatory surge.

Counter-Regulatory Hormones

During fasting, insulin falls; in response, other hormones, called *counter-regulatory hormones*, increase. This name derives from the fact that these hormones run counter, or opposite, to insulin. As insulin goes up, these counter-regulatory hormones go down. When insulin goes down, these hormones go up.

The effect on glucose metabolism is also opposite to one another. Insulin pushes the body toward *storage* of glucose and body fat, and counter-regulatory hormones push the body toward usage of glucose and body fat. The main counter-regulatory hormones that become elevated from the activation of the sympathetic nervous system include adrenaline and noradrenaline. Other counter-regulatory hormones are cortisol and growth hormone.

THE SYMPATHETIC NERVOUS SYSTEM

The sympathetic nervous system controls the so-called "fight or flight" response. For example, if you suddenly face a hungry lion, your body activates the sympathetic nervous system to prepare your body to fight or to run really, really fast.

Your pupils dilate, your heart rate increases, and your body pushes glucose into the blood for use as a ready source of energy. This is an extreme example; a milder form of sympathetic nervous system activation happens during the early fasting period. The hormones cortisol, adrenaline, and noradrenaline are released into the blood as part of the general activation of the body for action.

Contrary to many people's expectations, fasting, even for prolonged periods does not cause the body to shut down; instead, it ramps up and gets ready for action because of the energizing effect of the counter-regulatory hormones. Even up to four days of fasting results in an increase in resting energy expenditure (or basal metabolic rate).[6] This is the energy used to generate body heat and to fuel the brain, heart, liver, kidneys, and other organs. When measuring the energy used for metabolism, studies show that after four days of fasting the body is using 10 percent *more* energy than at the beginning of the fasting period. Although most people mistakenly believe that the body shuts down during fasting, the opposite is true. Fasting, at least up to four days, does not seem to make you tired; it gives you more energy.

During fasting, the body is merely switching fuel sources from food to stored food energy, also known as body fat. Imagine we are prehistoric men and women. It's winter, and food is scarce. We haven't eaten for four days. If our bodies begin to shut down, then it will be even harder to find food. We fall into a vicious cycle. Every day we don't eat means that it is much harder to get the energy to hunt or gather. As each day passes, our chance of survival progressively worsens. The human species would not have survived. Fortunately, our bodies are not that stupid.

Instead, our bodies switch fuel sources and pump us full of energy so that we have enough energy to hunt. Basal metabolism, sympathetic tone, and noradrenaline increase to fuel our bodies so that we can hunt. The VO2, a measure of the metabolic rate at rest, increases in conjunction.

GROWTH HORMONE

The other noteworthy counter-regulatory hormone that increases significantly during fasting periods is growth hormone (GH). Studies show that fasting for one day stimulates growth hormone secretion up to two to three times and continues to increase even up to five days of full fasting.[7] At first, this seems counterintuitive: Why would we want to increase growth at a time where we are not eating? Growth hormone does exactly what the name implies, telling the tissues of the body to grow bigger and taller. If there are no nutrients available, why grow?

We can find the answer by following our bodies through the entire feeding-fasting cycle. When we eat, glucose and amino acids are absorbed and transported to the liver. Insulin is secreted, telling the body to store the incoming food energy (calories). We are in the *fed* state. All tissues of the body use glucose, and the excess is stored in the liver as glycogen or as body fat.

Blood glucose and insulin fall several hours after a meal, signaling the start of the *fasted* state. As described earlier, the body goes through a predictable set of adaptations to fasting or starvation. Liver glycogen is mobilized and broken down to individual glucose for energy. Gluconeogenesis transforms some proteins into glucose. The body begins to shift from glucose metabolism to fat metabolism. During this time growth hormone is increasing, but no proteins are being synthesized because insulin and mTOR levels are low. So little growth is actually happening, despite the high GH levels.

Once you eat, or break the fast, the body goes into the fed state once again. After a long fast, growth hormone is high. Because amino acids are now plentiful after the meal, our bodies rebuild all the necessary proteins to replace those that were broken down. Insulin stimulates protein synthesis. So, now, in the refed state, the body has high insulin, high growth hormone, amino acids, and glucose for energy—all the components it needs to build or rebuild protein. As with autophagy, this process represents renewal, as the body breaks down unnecessary protein preferentially and rebuilds the most necessary ones. Fasting in this sense rejuvenates the lean tissues.

GLUCOSE REQUIREMENTS AND PROTEIN BREAKDOWN

Under conditions of fasting, the body must maintain sufficient glucose for normal brain functioning. Glucose requirements substantially lower as the liver and muscles switch to fatty acids, and the brain switches to ketones. The body can convert some of the glycerol from fatty acids to glucose, but there is a limit to the amount that can be converted. The rest of the glucose must be delivered by gluconeogenesis, so there is still a small amount of protein breakdown. However, the protein that's broken down is not specifically muscle cells. The proteins that turn over the most rapidly are the first proteins to be catabolized for glucose, including the skin and intestinal lining. In more than five years of working with patients in his Intensive Dietary Management program (www.IDMprogram.com), which uses therapeutic fasting for weight loss, Dr. Fung has not yet referred a patient for skin removal surgery—

even for those patients who have lost more than one hundred pounds. Immune cells also have a high turnover and might be reduced during fasting, which accounts for some of the anti-inflammatory effect seen clinically. Muscle cells, which turn over infrequently, are relatively spared. Overall, protein catabolism drops from approximately 75 grams per day to only 10 to 20 grams per day to preserve protein during prolonged starvation.[8]

There is a significant difference in protein metabolism between lean and obese subjects. During prolonged fasting, obese subjects burn two to three times less protein compared to lean subjects. This makes perfect sense. If people have more fat to burn, their bodies will use more of it. If there is less fat, the body is forced to rely on protein. This situation holds true not only for humans but also animals. More than one hundred years ago, researchers showed that the proportion of energy derived from protein was lower in animals with more body fat (mammals, geese) than in lean animals (rodents, dogs). If you have more fat, you use it before you use protein. Thus, although obese subjects have more overall protein than leaner subjects, the obese subjects lose it at a slower rate compared to leaner people (see Figure 7.3[9]).

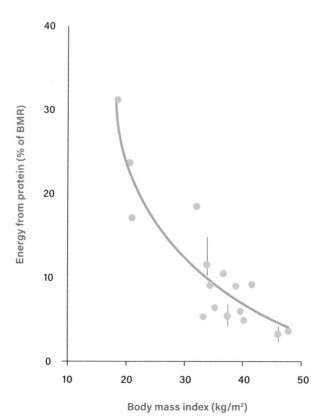

Fig. 7.3: Reduced protein breakdown during fasting with increasing Body Mass Index

During prolonged fasting, a person with a Body Mass Index of 20 (borderline underweight) derives almost 40 percent of energy needs from protein. Compare that to a person with a Body Mass Index of 50 (morbidly obese) who may derive only 5 percent of energy from protein stores (see the figure of reduced protein breakdown). Once again this demonstrates our body's inherent ability to survive. If we have stores of body fat, we use them. If we don't have those stores, we don't.

During prolonged fasting, fat oxidation accounts for approximately 94 percent of energy expenditure in obese subjects, whereas in lean subjects it's only 78 percent. Protein oxidation accounts for the remainder of the energy because there are almost no carbohydrate stores left in the body after the first twenty-four hours or so. Lean subjects also increase their ketone production much quicker than obese subjects.[10]

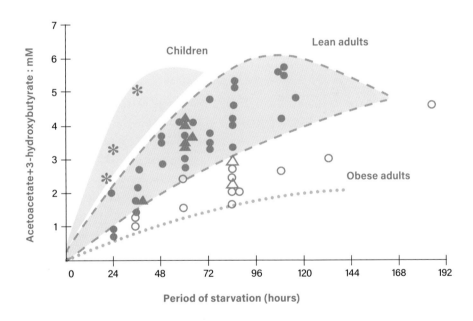

Fig. 7.4: Reduced protein breakdown during fasting with increasing Body Mass Index

> ## The difference in ketone production during starvation between children, lean adults, and obese adults.

Exactly how much protein you need during fasting depends upon your condition. If you're obese, fasting is very beneficial, and you will burn much more fat than protein. If you are quite lean, fasting might not be so beneficial because you will burn more protein. Your body is much smarter than you may give it credit for. It can handle itself during both feeding and fasting. Exactly how the body makes this adjustment is currently unknown.

Is this low level of protein breakdown a bad thing? Not necessarily. It is estimated that the obese person contains 50 percent more protein than a lean person.[11] All the excess skin, connective tissue holding up the fat cells, blood vessels to supply the extra bulk, and so on is made up of connective tissue. Think about a picture of a survivor of a Japanese prisoner of war camp in World War II. Is there any excess skin on that body? No, all that person's extra protein has been burned for energy or to maintain more important functions.

More importantly, many age-related diseases are characterized by excessive growth, not just of fat but also protein. Alzheimer's disease, for example, is characterized by the excessive accumulation of protein in the brain that blocks proper signaling. Cancer is excessive growth of many things, including many types of proteins. If many of the chronic diseases we face today are diseases of "too-much-growth," then the ability to break down proteins is a very powerful tool for health in the proper setting.

This may be the power of autophagy, the cellular recycling system that powerfully influences health. During fasting, which necessarily includes protein deprivation, the nutrient sensor mTOR is reduced, which stimulates the body to break down old, dysfunctional subcellular parts. Upon refeeding, the body builds new protein to replace the old in a complete renovation cycle. Instead of keeping old parts around, you are making new ones. Replacing old parts with new ones is an antiaging process.

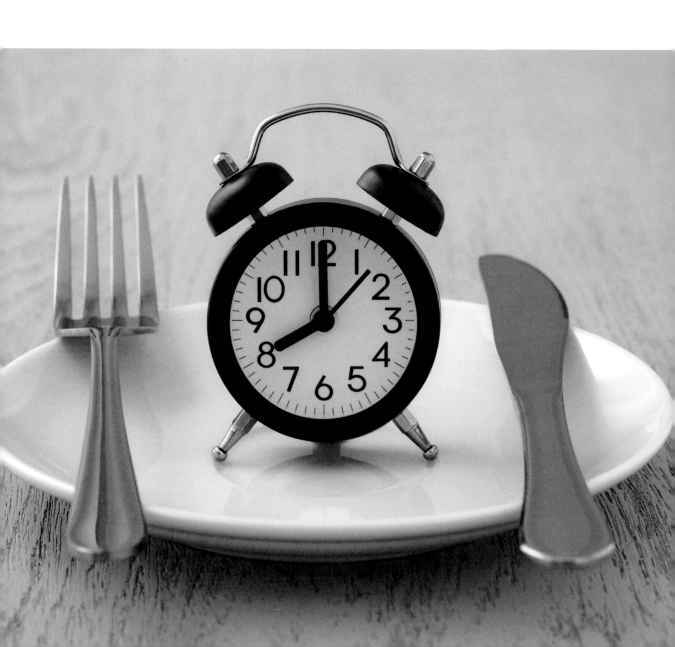

08

TEA

People of many cultures have been drinking tea for thousands of years. It has been used in many Asian cultures for its purported health benefits and as a way of bringing the family together. Tea is a complex brew that contains numerous longevity-promoting compounds. In this chapter, we discuss the history and health benefits of tea, as well as the compounds and mechanisms we believe give tea its health-promoting and longevity properties.

A Brief History

Tea is the second most popular beverage in the world; only water surpasses it. Tea drinking is thought to have originated in China. An estimated 2.5 million tons of tea leaves are produced annually, and approximately 20 percent of that is green tea. The oldest tree in existence, from the Yunnan province of China, is an estimated 3,200 years old.

According to legend, Shen Nong discovered tea in 2700 BC. He was trying to understand the effects of eating various plants, and he tasted more than one hundred plants in a single day. Shen Nong was boiling some water in a pot when some leaves fell in, and he discovered that tea had a bitter taste, but it could make his thoughts quicker and his vision clearer.

Tea drinking quickly went "viral" and would have broken the Internet had the Internet existed in 2700 BC. Explorers carried the practice of drinking tea throughout the world on the various ancient trade routes. Because unprocessed tea is quite bitter, the origins of the word *tea* come from *tu*, which means bitter. In the mid-seventh century, a stroke was removed from the original Chinese character, and the word became *cha*. Today, virtually all languages worldwide use variations of either *tea* or *cha*. The ancient Chinese Min Nan dialect of the Fujian province used the word *te*, which spread via sea trade and has been translated into all types of languages, from the English word *tea* to the Maori word *tii*. The dialects in landlocked regions of China used the word *cha* and spread tea via the ancient Silk Road; that term led to the Swahili *chai* and the Russian *chay*, for example.

Buddhist priests carried the tea-drinking tradition to Korea and Japan, where tea was believed to have many medicinal qualities. In 1211 AD, the Japanese Zen priest Yeisai published the book *Kitcha-Yojoki*, which translates to *Tea and Health Promotion*. He wrote about the harvesting and production of tea and its many healthful attributes. Yeisai proclaimed that tea was a "divine remedy and a supreme gift of heaven." Tea drinking had been restricted to nobility, but it started to spread to the general population. When the Shogun Sanetomo became ill from over-feasting, he summoned Yeisai to offer prayers. The priest supplemented his prayers with tea, and after the shogun recovered, he became a great tea devotee.

Portuguese traders brought tea from China to Europe, and by the 1600s it had spread to England; the English spread their cultural tastes (and their famous stiff upper lip) to much of the rest of the world. England bought so much tea from China that England developed a huge trade deficit because the Chinese didn't want any English products other than silver.

Arabs introduced opium to China around 400 AD. The English (and other Europeans) later exploited the situation by directing opium trade routes from India to China. The English increased opium trade in China purposely to create a nation of addicts and to help offset their trade deficit. The Chinese government was not happy about the burgeoning opioid crisis and moved to ban the trade. In true gangland, drug-pusher style, the English sent in their big gunships to make sure the opium flowed freely. Thus began the two Opium Wars that eventually won England the port of Hong Kong. As if that were not enough, the English then proceeded to smuggle some trees out of China to set up tea plantations in India, which broke China's 4,000-year-old monopoly on tea production. That's the kind of ruthlessness that wins you a global empire.

Early writings about tea focused on its medicinal effects, particularly for digestion, rather than the taste (bitter, kind of metallic). Most modern studies have focused on green tea because of the high concentration of polyphenols and the beneficial effects of a class of compounds called *catechins*, the most abundant of which is epigallocatechin-3-gallate (EGCG). According to traditional Chinese medicine, tea helps weight control, and current research may only now be catching up to this traditional way of thinking.

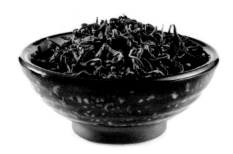

What Is Tea?

Tea is the leaf of the plant *Camellia sinensis*, an evergreen shrub native to Asia. The varieties we consume—white, green, pu-erh, oolong, and black—differ only by the processing. Freshly harvested leaves are steamed, rolled, and dried, which inactivates the enzymes responsible for breaking down the color; the result is the stable green tea leaves you can buy anywhere. The processing also helps preserve the natural polyphenols in the leaves.

White tea is entirely unfermented and is made by harvesting tea leaves before they are fully open, and tiny white hairs still cover the buds; hence the name *white tea*. Green tea is minimally fermented or not fermented at all. Pu-erh tea is made from a tea base called *maocha*, and then it's fermented, aged, and packed into tiny bricks; it has many flavors, including sweet, bitter, floral, mellow, woody, astringent, sour, earthy, watery, or even tasteless. Oolong tea is partially fermented, and full fermentation produces black tea. The polyphenols and catechins in unfermented tea change to theaflavins (although some EGCG metabolizes to theaflavins in the liver), which might have beneficial effects of their own, including antiviral, anticancer, and cholesterol-lowering benefits. People in Europe, North America, and North Africa drink mainly black tea, whereas Asians mostly drink oolong and green tea.

Tea contains more than 4,000 compounds, many of which appear to be beneficial for human health; the different classes of flavonoids are particularly beneficial. Other dietary sources of flavonoids include onions, apples, broccoli, and red wine, which is interesting because many of these foods are believed to be very healthy. An apple a day, for example, is purported to keep the doctor away. Red wine drinking has been associated with increased health and longevity. (Read more about red wine in Chapter 9.) Tea, which contains minerals, antioxidants, and amino acids, is one of the richest sources of phytonutrients available. The nations of East Asia, such as Japan, are among the largest drinkers of tea in the world. Perhaps not coincidentally, they also enjoy some of the highest life expectancies in the world.[1]

One cup of tea (2 grams dry tea leaves) provides 150 to 200 milligrams of flavonoids compared to an average daily flavonoid intake of less than 1,000 gm per day. A high intake of dietary flavonoids is associated with a 20 percent lower risk for heart disease.[2] Flavonoids may have a beneficial effect on the crucial endothelial cell layer that separates the blood from the artery wall. Any breach of this thin layer will expose the underlying blood vessel wall and trigger an inflammatory reaction that produces atherosclerosis (hardening of the arteries) and may even produce a blood clot, which is the underlying process of heart attacks and ischemic strokes. Depending on where this blockage occurs, this is called different things:

- In the heart, it's a heart attack.

- In the brain, it's an ischemic stroke.

- In the legs, it's peripheral vascular disease.

All types of blockages involve the same underlying damage to blood vessels and blood clots.

Studies of tea flavonoids[3] show significant improvements in endothelial health in both normal and diabetic populations. Flavonoids enhance the effect of nitric oxide (NO) a key molecule to relax blood vessels and lower blood pressure. Higher doses of black tea produce greater benefits. Researchers have noted similar benefits for flavonoids derived from chocolate and red wine.

In green tea, the main flavonoids are the colorless and water-soluble catechins that contribute to some of the bitterness and astringency of green tea. One cup of green tea contains 90 to 100 milligrams of catechins, and the catechins are potent antioxidants, which may help the body protect against inflammation. Green tea contains much higher concentrations of catechins than black teas; the catechins in green tea account for up to 30 percent of the dry weight. Furthermore, green tea is particularly high in one type of catechin—EGCG, which is responsible for 50 to 80 percent of total catechins in green tea. Standard brewing does not fully extract the catechins, so studies often use enriched green tea extracts (which are green teas that have been enriched with supplemental EGCG). Cold brewed green tea is another potential solution for fully extracting the catechins.

Catechins are absorbed in the intestine, but the presence of food significantly decreases their absorption. Consequently, drinking green tea on an empty stomach may increase catechin absorption. Because of the appetite-suppressing effects of green tea, some people might experience nausea. Hot brewed tea typically contains 70 to 100 grams of catechins. A cold brew crystal process (such as Pique tea crystals, https://www.picquetea.com) have about triple that amount of catechins per cup.

The Benefits of Tea on Disease

Various research studies have found that tea offers benefits for reducing the risk of various diseases, including cardiovascular disease, diabetes, cancer, and hypertension. The following sections describe some of the ways researchers have found tea to be beneficial.

CARDIOVASCULAR DISEASE

A large Dutch population study, called the European Prospective Investigation into Cancer and Nutrition (EPIC-NL)[4] followed 37,514 participants over 13 years and found that tea drinking was associated with less heart disease. Those who drank more than 6 cups per day had a 36 percent reduction in the incidence of heart disease. A 2001 meta-analysis suggested an 11 percent reduced risk of cardiovascular disease,[5] and the prospective 2002 Rotterdam study suggested that more than 375 milliliters per day (about 13 ounces or more) had a 70 percent lower risk![6]

The subjects in these European studies mostly drink black tea, but there is some evidence that green tea may be even more beneficial.[7] A meta-analysis suggests that moderate green tea consumption (one to three cups per day) is associated with a 19 percent reduced risk of heart disease, and drinking more than four cups per day increased that benefit to 32 percent. The prospective 2006 Ohsaki study also showed that drinking green tea is associated with strong protection against cardiovascular disease.[8] Over 11 years of follow up, the risk of death decreased by 15 percent, death from heart disease was down by 26 percent, and death from stroke was reduced by 37 percent, as shown in Figure 8.1.

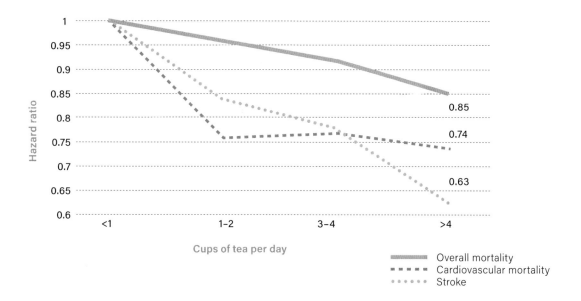

Fig. 8.1: Ohsaki study results

There may be some important differences between the types of tea (green versus black) and the style of tea drinking. In North America, people often buy tea from the coffee shop, paying $1.50 or so for a tea bag and some hot water. If you drink six cups per day, as some subjects have done in some of these studies, you'd have to pay $9 per day.

However, in Asia where people drink tea like water, a teapot full of tea leaves was steeped over and over again. Whenever a person is thirsty, they would pour some tea. At restaurants, it's the same thing. When people go out for lunch in Hong Kong, *yum cha* literally means "to drink tea." A pot of tea stays on the table, and the waiter keeps refilling it with hot water as needed for everybody to enjoy throughout the entire meal. At many homes, people do the same. Instead of getting glasses of water with dinner, the family might refill the teapot and drink some hot tea. In Asia, tea is the default drink throughout the day, and therefore you can easily drink six or eight cups a day without even thinking about it. North Americans might drink six to eight glasses of water instead, although that's the best-case scenario. Many North American children drink sugary sodas or fruit juices instead.

There's another important difference in tea drinking traditions between the East and West. In Asia, tea is usually taken straight, without any added sugar or milk. In the United Kingdom, it is estimated that 99 percent of tea drinkers add milk to their tea. Does the added milk make a difference? The Caerphilly study[9] from South Wales found no reduction in heart disease with increased tea drinking, in contrast to other studies mentioned earlier. Researchers speculated that milk blocked the absorption of flavonoids from the tea. Experimental evidence shows that the antioxidant effect of both green and black tea was completely inhibited by adding milk. Proteins in milk form complexes with polyphenols that might block absorption.[10]

The benefits of drinking straight tea also extend to the prevention of stroke.[11] A 2009 meta-analysis showed that people who drank three or more cups of tea per day had a 21 percent reduced risk of stroke. In addition to improving endothelial function and lowering blood pressure, tea contains theanine. Tea leaves have a high concentration of this amino acid, and dietary theanine comes almost exclusively from that source. Theanine easily crosses the blood-brain barrier and might help protect against damage from stroke.

OBESITY AND TYPE 2 DIABETES

Since 1977, obesity and type 2 diabetes have become a worldwide epidemic. Prevention and treatment strategies have become global priorities.

Many miracle diet pills have come and gone. The notorious Fen-Phen, a prescription medication, was like the old street drug "speed" in that it caused weight loss by speeding up metabolism, but it also caused all kinds of heart problems. Fen-Phen could make you thin, but it also could kill you. Orlistat was another drug that blocked fat absorption. It caused weight loss, but it had some bothersome side effects like diarrhea from malabsorption of fat. The best advice for someone taking Orlistat was not to wear white pants. Then there was sibutramine, which caused weight loss, but side effects like heart attacks and strokes caused it to be discontinued.

There were weight loss supplements that wouldn't kill you, but they didn't work. Green coffee bean extract, raspberry ketones, and grapefruit extract all come to mind. They sound great, but they all turned out to be pure hype.

However, there's one substance that seems to have stood the test of time: green tea. Traditional Asian medicine has touted the weight loss effects of green tea for thousands of years.

A 2016 randomized trial showed that high-dose green tea extract (EGCG 856 milligrams) significantly reduced weight by more than 1 kilogram, and it also reduced waist circumference.[12] In tea drinkers, the hunger hormone ghrelin also was significantly reduced by the catechins when compared to non-tea drinkers. Obviously, hunger control leads to easier weight loss.

Hunger is one of the most powerful human needs, and controlling hunger is one of the keys to long-term weight loss. Most calorie restriction plans ignore this factor and pretend that willpower is more important. You can't "decide" to be less hungry. You can temporarily ignore hunger, but when it persists day after day, it is impossible to ignore. Green tea, with its small effect on decreasing ghrelin, is a great complement to fasting, and both are important components of longevity. However, the dose of catechins used in the study would require you to drink twelve cups of hot brewed green tea per day.

A 2009 meta-analysis also found similar benefits to green tea drinking, with an average loss of 1.31 kilograms of body weight.[13] The catechins in green tea may help with weight loss by increasing the metabolic rate.[14] A beverage containing green tea catechins and caffeine increased the daily energy expenditure by an average of 106 calories per day, or 4.6 percent. This effect was likely due to both the catechins and caffeine in green tea. However, green tea performed 50 to 100 percent better than expected compared to caffeine alone. Other studies[15] found an almost identical 4 percent increase in metabolic rate even in tests of half the amount of caffeine. It was noted in a Cochrane review[16] that the benefits were not seen when brewed green tea was used; the results occurred only with the catechin-enriched tea.

Oolong tea may also show this benefit, with studies demonstrating that consuming five 10-ounce servings per day for three days raises energy expenditure by 2.9 percent (about 67 calories) and fat oxidation by 12 percent.[17] Oolong tea is semifermented and thus represents a sort of medium ground between green and black tea. It is very popular in China and Japan.

Green tea promotes long-term weight loss by increasing basal metabolic rate, improving glucose uptake by muscle, and enhancing fat-burning in the liver and muscle.[18] Although the effects on basal metabolic rate are not huge, we don't win the battle for weight loss by creating a small caloric deficit; we win by improving the overall metabolic health of the body. Thus, although the difference of burning an extra 100 calories per day might not be very significant, an improvement in glucose and fat burning (and a reduction in hunger) is what makes the difference. It's like taking out an old engine and putting in a brand-new V10 engine. You are a better fat- and glucose-burning machine. And fat loss is about enhancing your body's metabolic machinery because that determines what your body does with the calories you eat (either storing them or burning them); it's not about creating a small deficit of calories. All these beneficial effects make tea drinking a highly effective intervention for health.

Because obesity and type 2 diabetes are closely linked, we might expect that the weight-loss benefits with tea and tea catechins also could translate into benefits for type 2 diabetes. Indeed, that appears to be exactly the case. A 2009 placebo-controlled trial[19] showed spectacular results. Green tea enriched with 582.8 milligrams of catechins reduced hemoglobin A1C (a marker for three-month average blood glucose levels) by 0.37. That result is almost as powerful as some of the medications used today for treatment of diabetes. The waist circumference, which is indicative of the more dangerous abdominal fat, was reduced by 3.3 cm. Systolic blood pressure was reduced by 5.9 mmHg and diastolic by 3.0 mmHg; triglycerides improved by more than 10 percent.

The 2006 Japan Collaborative Cohort Study for Evaluation of Cancer Risk[20] followed more than 16,000 subjects and found that drinking green tea (six or more cups per day versus less than one cup per week) was associated with a 33 percent decreased risk for developing type 2 diabetes. Researchers found no association between consumption of black and oolong teas and the risk for diabetes. The MEDIS study[21] of 1,190 elderly patients in Greece, Cyprus, and Crete also found that moderate (one to two cups), long-term (at least thirty years) consumption of green or black tea was significantly associated with lower blood glucose and 70 percent lower odds of having type 2 diabetes. Interestingly, almost all of the tea drinkers in the study were also coffee drinkers, which suggests additional benefits even on top of coffee consumption.

Asians show consistently better results compared to Caucasians, which is perhaps a result of genetic differences. Catechins inhibit the enzyme COMT, which increases energy expenditure. Asians have higher rates of the high-activity COMT(H), so blocking it with green tea catechins would be predicted to show greater effects, explaining the racial difference. Weight loss for Asians averaged 1.51 kilograms, but only 0.8 kilogram for Caucasians. However, 0.8 kilogram is still a substantial benefit.[22]

HYPERTENSION

High blood pressure (hypertension) has been called the silent killer because it increases the risk of heart disease and stroke, yet there often are few symptoms. Traditional Chinese medicine believes that tea reduces blood pressure and modern studies confirm this assertion. A Norwegian study[23] showed that drinking tea was associated with lower blood pressure even after twelve years of follow up. The effect was moderate (4 mmHg), but when this effect is combined with an improvement in endothelial function[24] and is multiplied by millions of men and women over decades, the overall effect is huge, and the potential savings in both money and human suffering is massive. A Taiwanese study showed similar results.[25] The study showed the same dose-response relationship, but it also showed that those who habitually drank tea for many years had lower blood pressures.

Green tea may also have many of these antihypertensive benefits. A 2011 randomized trial[26] showed a 5 mmHg drop in blood pressure. However, there also were improvements in cholesterol (lower LDL, higher HDL), insulin resistance, inflammation, and oxidative stress.

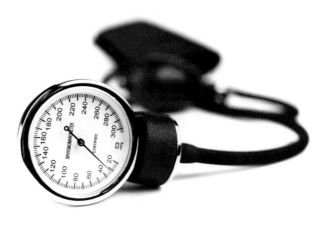

CANCER

There is inconsistent data on the effect of tea on cancer. According to the National Cancer Institute, "The results of these studies have often been inconsistent, but some have linked tea consumption to reduced risks of cancers of the colon, breast, ovary, prostate, and lung."[27] The main catechin in green tea, EGCG, has been shown to be an inhibitor of both mTOR and the PI3K growth pathway that is stimulated by insulin. Both pathways are overactive in many cancers, so regular drinking of green tea might help prevent cancers.

Drinking tea may potentially improve cancer outcomes and reduce the risk for breast cancer.[28] Breast cancer recurrence and colorectal cancer may both be reduced in regular green tea drinkers.[29] The catechins in green tea might help prevent metastasis or induced apoptosis (programmed cell death). EGCG binds to the death ligand to activate the mitochondrial pathway. Once activated, the cell dies and never has a chance to become cancerous.

Why Drink Tea?

Because tea is so widely consumed, the potential for changing health is immense. Even if there exists only a small benefit for tea, when multiplied by billions of people drinking it multiple times per day, it can add up to substantial benefits for public health. There are substantial data suggesting benefits for weight loss and lower risk of heart disease, stroke, cancer, and type 2 diabetes. Tea contributes in many different ways to longevity and has been a part of human culture for many millennia.

The bottom line is relatively simple. There are many potential benefits with virtually no risks, and the cost for this form of prevention is low. Drinking tea comes with a very high benefit-to-risk ratio, so the better question is "Why would you *not* drink tea?"

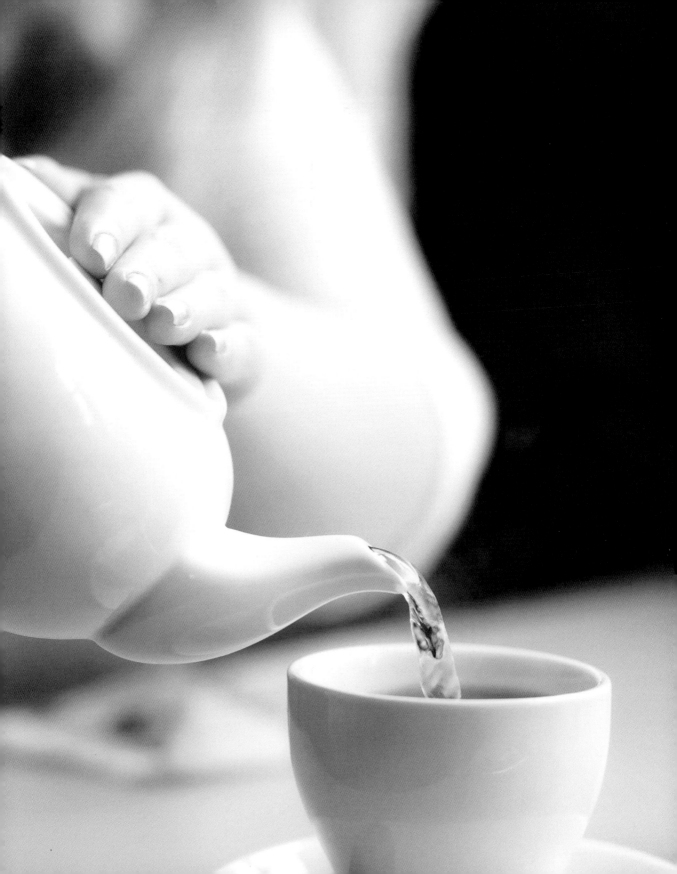

09
RED WINE AND COFFEE

The history of wine-making dates back more than 10,000 years to when it was discovered in Caucasia before it spread to Mesopotamia, Phoenicia, Egypt, Greece, and the Mediterranean.[1] Wine was initially revered worldwide as a source of longevity and health, but later it became better known as a deadly toxin, and many countries banned it during Prohibition. In the last fifty years, the viewpoint has been shifting back in the direction of considering it to be a healthy habit to drink some wine. Science is only now catching up to what ancient civilizations long knew. In this chapter, we discuss the health benefits of consuming red wine and coffee and tell you how much of each beverage you should be consuming per day.

Red Wine

The Hunza valley lies in the Himalayan Mountains of northern Pakistan, 8,500 feet above sea level. The Hunza people, who are completely isolated from other civilizations by the surrounding mountain peaks, are famous for their longevity. In 1979, visiting scholars were astounded[2] by several centenarians who ranged in age from 101 to 109 and were seemingly in perfect health. They had normal blood pressures, and electrocardiogram (EKG) testing revealed no recognizable atherosclerosis. They were agile for their age; not only could they walk and move about effortlessly but their favorite hobby was going out and working the nearby terraced fields. This lifestyle differs markedly from the elderly in the United States. If Americans are lucky enough to reach the age of 100, they're often barely able to walk to the bathroom. There is some controversy about the Hunza citizens' actual ages because there were no birth certificates, but they nonetheless had clearly managed to age gracefully.

The Hunza prize the locally grown apricots and add them to their homemade wine, which is called *Hunza-Pani* (or "Hunza water"). Six of the remarkable centenarians said that they drank wine every day. At feasts, the Hunza freely drink their homemade wine. They consider it their secret for longevity and stress relief,[3] and it could be yours too.

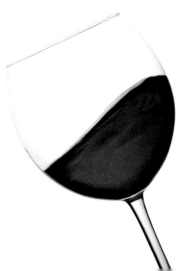

RED WINE THROUGHOUT HISTORY

> *"Wine is an appropriate article for mankind, both for the healthy body and for the ailing man."*

—Hippocrates

Wine has been part of human culture for thousands of years, not only as part of our diet but also part of our social and religious history. It predates Biblical times at least to the Neolithic period (approximately 10,000 BC), but it was almost certainly consumed much earlier. Alcohol was produced in practically every part of the world, differing only by what was used to make it. But was this elixir healthy, or was it harmful?

Hippocrates, the father of modern medicine, believed that men should live on large quantities of "watered wine."[4] It was commonplace to mix wine with water to prevent overt intoxication. Sometimes wine was sweetened with honey. Hippocrates recommended wine as a disinfectant on wounds and even prescribed wine as a tranquilizer, an analgesic, and a diuretic.[5] The ancient Greeks used wine as both food and medicine. They washed wounds with wine and used it as a medium for taking medicine.[6]

The Greeks and the Romans believed the consumption of low doses of wine was beneficial to many aspects of health. The Greek physician Rufus of Ephesus, in the first century AD, wrote, "Wine is more praiseworthy for health than any other thing; however, anyone who drinks it must be wise, if he does not wish to suffer some irreparable ill."[7] This captures the essential dual nature of alcohol. In small doses, it can be highly beneficial, but it is toxic in large doses.

In ancient Rome, Caesar ordered his soldiers to drink wine with meals to protect against gastrointestinal infections.

Paracelsus, a German doctor practicing in the sixteenth century, wrote, "Whether wine is a nourishment, medicine, or poison is a matter of dosage." Paracelsus is considered the father of toxicology and is credited with creating the essential rule, "The dose makes the poison." The use of smaller doses of "toxic" substances for health is called *hormesis*. Some examples of toxic substances we use to promote health include botulinum toxin (Botox) and rat poison (Coumadin, used for thinning the blood). The principle also might apply to red wine.

Even Thomas Jefferson wrote, "Wine of long habit has become indispensable to my health." Famous French biologist Louis Pasteur wrote that he found "wine to be the most healthful and hygienic of beverages." And in the writings in which William Heberden described angina pectoris, he noted "wines and spirituous liquors afford considerable relief"; he believed that wine was a potent coronary vasodilator.[8]

However, this attitude that red wine was a factor in longevity and important for maintaining good cardiovascular health changed dramatically in the early twentieth century as public opinion embraced the idea that alcohol was toxic in any dose. This culminated in Prohibition in many nations of the world, including the United States from 1920 to 1933.

During Prohibition, all sales, transportation, and drinking of alcohol were banned. The leaders of the Prohibition movement were concerned about the many problems associated with alcoholism, including health problems, such as liver cirrhosis, and numerous social problems, like domestic violence and absenteeism. The temperance movement began in the early nineteenth century, but it gained strength with The Anti-Saloon League, which formed in 1893. Prohibition planted the idea that a complete ban on alcohol and related businesses would be a great boon to public health.

Alcohol consumption did indeed dramatically fall in 1920, with estimates that per-capita alcohol use dropped by about 30 percent. But further reductions were impossible because of illegal imports, moonshine, and organized crime. Prohibition finally was repealed; however, it left the impression among the public that all alcohol was bad for health. Abstinence was considered a virtue, and this viewpoint persisted through the rest of the twentieth century.

Improbably, as we moved into the twenty-first century, studies consistently found that moderate alcohol consumption reduced heart disease. Red wine provided the greatest protection.[9] However, consuming large amounts of alcohol is a slippery slope because higher amounts are still associated with greater mortality and higher risk for heart failure and arrhythmias. The dose makes the poison.

THE FRENCH PARADOX: IS RED WINE THE SECRET INGREDIENT?

Since the 1960s Americans have believed that eating too much fat would cause heart disease. In a desperate attempt to expunge fat from our diet, we cut the visible fat off meat, ate low-fat skinless chicken breasts, and drank low-fat dairy. Meanwhile, citizens of France continued to enjoy their traditional full-fat cheeses and fatty cuts of meat. The French ate almost three times as much of the reviled animal fats compared to Americans but had almost half the heart disease.[10] We call this "The French Paradox,"[11] although it could easily apply to people in Greece or Spain who also consume diets relatively high in saturated fat but have a low rate of death from heart disease. Much of this "paradox" is explained by the fact that natural animal fats don't cause heart disease, which is an understanding that is still evolving. We address types of fats in more detail in Chapter 11.

Scientific investigation into this paradox led researchers onto a surprising new path to uncovering the benefits of red wine. The French Paradox is unique because of the much higher rate at which the French consume alcohol compared to the people of other countries.[12] France produces more wine than any other country in the world and ranks second in the number of vineyards (just behind Spain). Although red wine was previously thought to be a risk factor for heart disease, it increasingly is viewed as a protective factor.

The first inklings of the surprising notion that low-moderate alcohol intake could be beneficial came in 1979. Researchers surveyed eighteen developed countries, including Canada and the United States, to look for factors related to heart disease deaths.[9] The researchers were not interested in wine at all. Instead, their main interest was the correlation between the number of doctors and nurses and improved health care for the patient. Surprisingly, countries with more doctors also had more heart disease. Because the research also included information about health and alcohol use, the researchers were able to examine outcomes related to alcohol consumption. For example, increased alcohol intake was associated with more road accident deaths, which underscores the importance of not drinking and driving.

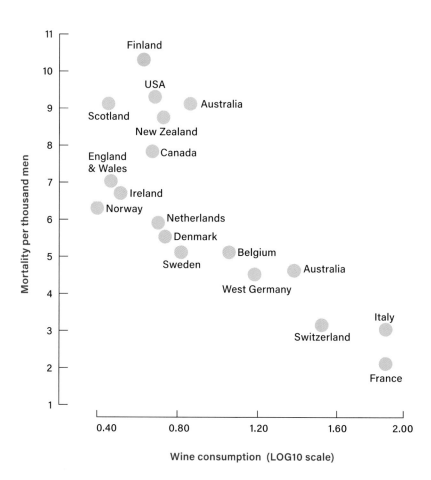

Fig. 9.1: Wine consumption and cardiac death in developed countries[13]

The researchers uncovered that the most powerful protective factor against heart disease was moderate alcohol consumption, which was a completely unexpected result. As they looked further into the phenomenon by separating wine, beer, and spirits, researchers found that the protective effect occurred only in the wine drinkers.

Since this study, many other studies have confirmed this unanticipated finding, proving that the results were no fluke.

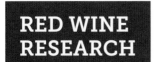

RED WINE RESEARCH The Copenhagen city heart study followed almost 20,000 individuals for twelve years;[14] once again, moderate daily intake of alcohol was associated with less risk of death (see Figure 9.2). As in the 1979 study, the positive effect was limited to wine and was not observed with either beer or spirits.

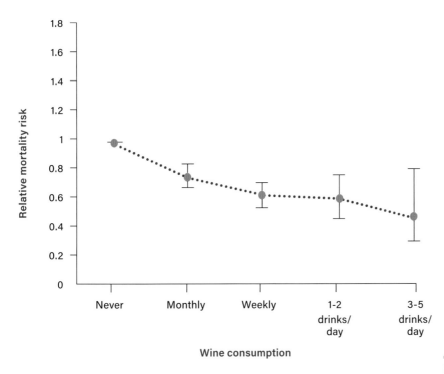

Fig. 9.2: The relationship of relative mortality risk and wine consumption

The benefits of drinking wine were not trivial. People who drank three to five drinks per day died at a rate almost *half* those who never drank wine (relative risk 0.51). That's a stunning benefit.

A French study showed that moderate alcohol intake was associated with a 33 percent reduced risk of death from all causes but showed no benefit for beer.[15] In China, where alcohol intake is primarily from rice wine, a study noted a smaller but still significant 19 percent reduction in risk of death.[16] Data from the Cancer Prevention Study II, which covered almost 1.2 million

Americans, revealed a 30 to 40 percent lower risk of death with moderate alcohol use (see the following graph). The greatest benefits occurred with one drink per day. Excessive alcohol use was still found to be dangerous, particularly in younger people, for whom there was an increased risk of violent deaths and accidents. Excessive alcohol in older people increased the risk of liver cirrhosis.[17]

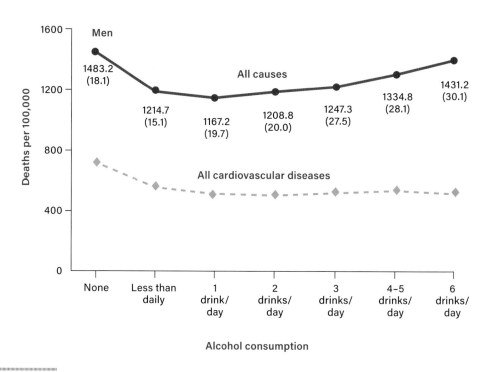

Fig. 9.3: Alcohol consumption and mortality

Other studies corroborated what was found in the Cancer Prevention Study II by showing a lower risk of all-cause mortality and coronary heart disease with moderate alcohol consumption (see Figure 9.4).

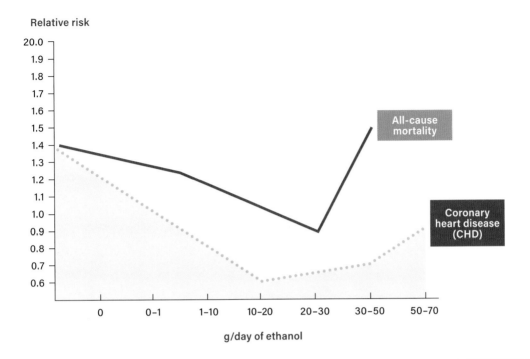

Relative risk

g/day of ethanol

Fig. 9.4: Alcohol, particularly red wine, may decrease the risk of coronary heart disease and death[18]

Data from the United States shows what you might expect. Moderate alcohol reduces cardiovascular disease, but further drinking does not increase the benefits. Drinking more alcohol increased the risk of alcohol-augmented conditions, including liver disease and certain cancers, which negates some of the beneficial effects. In military recruits, greater alcohol consumption increased the risk of death, mostly from accidents, suicide, and violence.[19]

Most recently, the Women's Health Study demonstrated once again that, compared to no alcohol use, moderate drinking was associated with a 35 percent reduced risk of overall death and a 51 percent reduced risk of cardiovascular death.[20] One of the longest studies, the Zutphen study, followed 1,373 men over 40 years. This study found that, compared to abstinence, moderate drinking (about a half glass per day) might prolong life by five years![21]

It is important to note that many of these studies examine daily alcohol intake rather than binge drinking. Drinking one to two glasses of wine daily with dinner is different from drinking four bottles once a week. Context is vitally important. Alcohol is a powerful weapon in the fight for longevity, but, like any weapon, it cuts both ways. Used poorly and without knowledge, it will hurt the user.

Consume red wine with food

One reason why studies in the United States have not shown results as impressive as European studies is that Europeans almost always consume their wine with dinner, which is not always the case in the United States. Americans tend to drink socially, whereas our European counterparts view wine as part of the meal. Drinking red wine with a meal maximizes one of the main health benefits of the wine, which is its ability to decrease after-meal spikes in lipids and glucose. Drinking red wine with a meal decreases the amount and time that VLDL, cholesterol remnant particles, and glucose come in contact with your blood vessels. These particles can cause damage to the endothelium and promote endothelial dysfunction, which can lead to hypertension and atherosclerosis in the arteries.

MECHANISMS OF BENEFIT

Wine contains approximately 12 to 15 percent alcohol by volume. Alcohol itself might have some healthy effects, but more likely it's the other bioactive compounds in red wine that are responsible for the benefits. Polyphenols in red wine potentially reduce the clotting tendency of blood and reduce LDL oxidation (see Figure 9.5).[22]

Fig. 9.5: The benefits of plant flavonoids

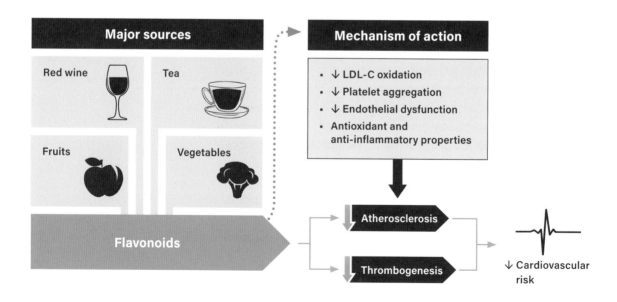

Red wine, and alcohol in general, beneficially affects cholesterol, particularly raising high-density lipoprotein, known as HDL or "good" cholesterol (see Figure 9.6).[23]

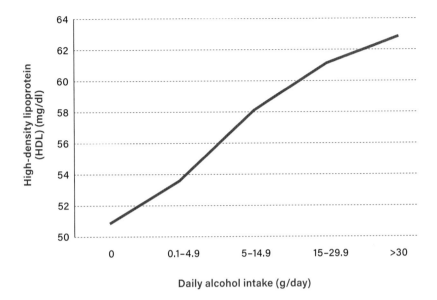

Fig. 9.6: Alcohol intake and HDL levels

Wine, as well as some other alcoholic beverages and tea, contains biologically active constituents called *polyphenols*. Red wine is produced from the entire grape, including the skin and seed, whereas white wine is produced after the skin has been removed. Red wine is macerated with the skin and seeds for several weeks, and this results in up to ten times the amount of polyphenols depending upon the specifics of the type of grape and its specific fermentation process. Red wines contain 750 to 1060 milligrams per liter of flavonoids compared to 25 to 30 milligrams in white wines.[24]

One polyphenol is exclusive to red wine: *resveratrol*. Resveratrol comes from grape skins, so the only significant dietary source of this polyphenol comes from red wine.[20] Since its discovery, many supplement companies rushed to make resveratrol tablets. Unfortunately, the supplements were not effective at promoting health because resveratrol is absorbed in the body only when it is ingested as wine. At concentrations found after consuming red wine, resveratrol can increase endothelial nitric oxide synthase and promotes an increase in nitric oxide (NO). Nitric oxide is a biological gas, which dilates the arteries, prevents atherosclerosis, and protects against blood clots due to its antiplatelet effects. Polyphenols can act as potent antioxidants and reduce platelet clumping and thus thin the blood and relax the blood vessels through endothelial NO release. Resveratrol prolongs life in yeast by activation of the longevity gene Sirt1, the same gene implicated for the effect of calorie restriction. For this reason, Sirtuins are known as "the enzymes of youth."[25]

Moderate alcohol consumption also reduces inflammation, blood clotting,[26] and blood pressure.[27] A meta-analysis of fifteen human studies estimated that alcohol consumption reduced the systolic blood pressure (the top number) by 3.31 mmHg and the diastolic blood pressure by 2.04 mmHg.[28] Although these reductions seem rather small, the benefit is greater than the reduction researchers observed with salt restriction, and that reduction launched a vicious fifty-year attack on salt. Just like salt, moderate alcohol intake is associated with less heart disease, not more.

High insulin levels and insulin resistance are the core causes of metabolic syndrome, which substantially raises the risk of future heart disease and stroke. The Normative Aging Study from Harvard University,[29] including its 30 years of follow-up, discovered that moderate intake of alcohol was associated with significantly lower insulin levels and insulin resistance than either the high-intake or no-alcohol group. In 2005, the American Diabetes Association found a highly significant 30 percent reduction in type 2 diabetes with moderate drinking.[30] Researchers estimated that the reduction in heart disease deaths with moderate alcohol was largely attributable to the following things:

- Improved cholesterol profiles
- Improved blood glucose/diabetes[31]
- Improvement in inflammation/blood clotting
- Blood pressure reduction

The remaining benefits of alcohol are largely through unknown mechanisms.

How much red wine should you drink?

The 2015–2020 Dietary Guidelines for Americans recommend moderate consumption of alcohol (two drinks per day for men and one drink per day for women). A standard drink is defined as 14 grams of pure ethanol. A meta-analysis of fifty-one studies indicates that consuming around 12.5 grams of alcohol per day is associated with the lowest risk for coronary heart disease for women, and 25 grams in men.[32] For most red wines, which are around 12.5 percent ethanol, about 3 ounces of red wine per day may be optimal for women, and 6 ounces of red wine per day for men. For people who are in certain high-risk situations, such as children, women who are pregnant or breastfeeding, alcoholics, and those taking medications that interact with alcohol, this recommendation does not apply, and you should avoid alcohol.

Six red wine tips

1. Drink red wine with meals. This decreases blood glucose levels[34] and prevents blood pressure increases that may happen when alcohol is taken alone.

2. Marinate meats in red wine before cooking. This decreases the formation of carcinogenic chemicals (heterocyclic amines) that might be formed with high-heat cooking.

3. French and Brazilian red wines, pinot noir, and Lambrusco are great choices. They have the highest concentrations of resveratrol and polyphenols that may protect the heart and brain.

4. If you can't drink alcohol, try de-alcoholized red wine, which may have similar benefits.

5. Drink moderate amounts daily and avoid binge drinking.[33]

6. Many wines contain loads of added sugar, so it's important to consume a low-sugar wine, such as those from Dry Farm Wines (www.dryfarmwines.com). Here are some advantages of Dry Farm Wines: They're sugar free, mold free, and gluten free; they're low in sulfites; they have no additives; and they have a low alcohol content (less than 12.5%).

Coffee

The story of coffee dates back to the ancient coffee forests of Ethiopia.[35] Legend tells of a goat herder named Kaldi who discovered coffee when he noticed that some of his goats became energetic and would not sleep at night after eating the berries from a certain tree. The berries were turned into a drink, and people discovered that it provided energy and alertness. And so coffee cultivation was born. The trade of coffee first became popular in the Arabian Peninsula, and by the sixteenth century coffee had spread to Persia, Egypt, Syria, and Turkey. By the seventeenth century, coffee had made its way to Europe; shortly after, it spread to the rest of the world.[36]

BENEFITS OF COFFEE

In the United States, coffee is the second-most widely consumed beverage (after water) and the main source of caffeine intake among adults. Coffee is a complex beverage containing more than 1,000 compounds, many with known biological activity, such as caffeine, diterpene alcohols, chlorogenic acid, lignans, and trigonelline. It's the single largest source of antioxidants in the American diet. A typical 8-ounce cup of coffee contains anywhere from 95 to 200 milligrams of caffeine, whereas decaffeinated coffee contains only 5 to 15 milligrams of caffeine per 8 ounces.[37] The caffeine content of coffee may play a role in delivering some of its health benefits.

Coffee consumption is associated with a lower risk for type 2 diabetes mellitus.[38] Coffee reduces two-hour post-glucose challenge blood sugar levels by an average of 13.1 percent[39] and reduces hemoglobin A1C (a measure of overall glucose exposure) by 7.5 percent. Waist circumference, a key indicator of metabolic syndrome, significantly decreased, but only in the caffeinated coffee group. When a person consumes 300 milligrams of caffeine per day, their energy expenditure increases by 80 kilocalories per day,[40] which may have been enough to account for the difference in waist circumference. Although caffeine can acutely decrease insulin sensitivity in humans,[41] the effects over a longer term seem beneficial.

Two large meta-analyses confirm an inverse relationship between coffee intake and the risk of type 2 diabetes, and they demonstrate the clear dose-response relationship. Drinking more coffee lowers the risk of type 2 diabetes.[42] Drinking four to six cups of coffee daily is associated with a 28 percent reduction in the risk of developing type 2 diabetes, whereas drinking more than six cups shows a 35 percent reduction. A large Japanese study with thirteen years of follow-up found a 42 percent decreased risk of type 2 diabetes in people who drink coffee frequently.[43]

Although coffee might be beneficial, what people add to the coffee (cream and sugar) is not so benign. As Dr. DiNicolantonio and two other colleagues have said, "If looking for longevity, say yes to the coffee, no to the sugar."[44]

There are other benefits to coffee drinking. Drinking five cups of instant caffeinated or decaffeinated coffee improved adipocyte and liver function, respectively, via changes in adiponectin and fetuin-A concentrations.[45] Drinking two to five cups (16 to 40 ounces) of coffee per day is associated with lower rates of mortality, death from cardiovascular disease, type 2 diabetes, liver disease, Parkinson's, depression, and suicide.[46]

A large Dutch population study called the European Prospective Investigation into Cancer and Nutrition (EPIC-NL)[47] followed 37,514 participants over thirteen years with food frequency questionnaires (see Figure 9.7). Those who drank moderate amounts of coffee had modest protection against heart disease. However, drinking more than six cups of coffee per day seemed to attenuate some of those benefits. This data is more or less in line with results from other studies that indicate moderate coffee drinking (three to four cups) might have some potential benefits.

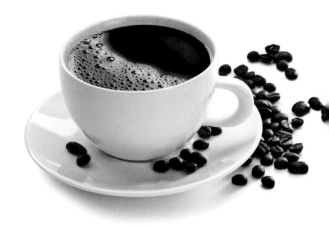

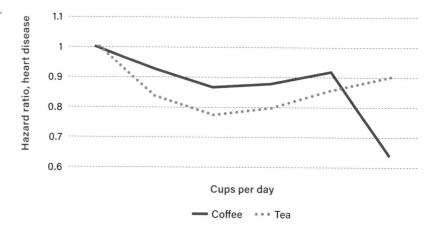

Fig. 9.7: Cardiac protection with tea and coffee (EPIC-NL)

In one of the most comprehensive reviews on the subject, Poole and colleagues concluded that consuming three to four cups of coffee per day was associated with the largest benefit for reducing all-cause mortality, cardiovascular mortality, and cardiovascular disease.[48] This also included an 18 percent lower risk of cancer, with no evidence of harmful associations. European studies also found that heavy coffee drinkers had a 22 percent lower risk of all-cause mortality.[49] An analysis of three large prospective cohorts found that drinking one to five cups of coffee per day was associated with a significantly lower risk of mortality with evidence of a dose-response relationship.[50]

ADD HONEY TO YOUR COFFEE

To add a little natural sweetness to your coffee, you can add some raw honey. Rainforest1st Wild Tualang Honey appears to be the only available FDA-certified raw tualang honey (www.rainforest1st.com). Tualang honey is a very dark honey, which generally contains more antioxidants and nutrients compared to lighter honeys. The darker the honey, the better it is for your health.

MECHANISMS OF BENEFITS

Coffee is a rich source of chlorogenic acid, which is metabolized to caffeic acid and then ferulic acid in the body. Blood levels of ferulic acid are even higher than caffeic acid in the hours following coffee consumption,[51] and this may drive many of the health benefits. In rodents, ferulic acid is protective against Parkinson's disease[52] and also increases the synthesis of the antioxidant glutathione.[53] Ferulic acid can act as a scavenger, stabilizer, and chain-breaker of free radicals due to its phenolic nucleus and its highly conjugated structure, which may help to protect against UV radiation and lipid peroxidation.[54] Ferulic acid also has been noted to protect against cerebral ischemia-reperfusion injury,[55] and it reduces the harm from the inflammatory cytokine TNF-alpha.[56]

POTENTIAL SIDE EFFECTS OF COFFEE

Potential adverse effects of caffeinated coffee may include insomnia, increased urination and thirst, dehydration, palpitations, and tremors. In the elderly, bone loss is a potential adverse effect.[57] Caffeine is a diuretic and can cause an increased loss of sodium, chloride, and calcium from the urine.[58] Each cup of coffee causes an additional 437 milligrams of urinary sodium loss, so drinking four cups of coffee would require eating an extra half teaspoon of salt to replace those losses.[59]

Consuming coffee and caffeine during pregnancy can increase the risk of preterm labor and low birth weight. Also, drinking coffee on a regular basis can lead to physical and psychological dependence. However, dependence might be an advantageous side effect because it helps to reinforce daily consumption of coffee, which is associated with a broad range of health benefits.

10

EAT MORE SALT AND MAGNESIUM

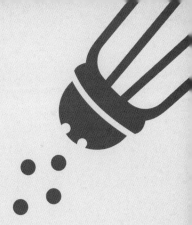

We think of salt more like a poison than an essential mineral. The Dietary Guidelines, health agencies, and doctors tell us that the lower the salt intake, the better. But does any real evidence support this notion? Where does the idea that salt is bad for us come from? In this chapter, we review the key players in the history of the low-salt dogma and show how eating more salt can actually improve your health.

Like salt, magnesium is an important mineral. However, unlike the heavy clouds hovering over the white crystal, magnesium has a health halo—and for good reason. Magnesium is vital for more than 600 reactions in the body, and many of us are being depleted of magnesium due to lifestyle choices, chronic diseases, and medications. Salt and magnesium are intricately connected, which is a relationship long forgotten. In the following pages, we explain the benefits of magnesium, what factors cause its deficiency, and which forms of magnesium are the best for supplementation.

Low-Salt Advice: Clear, Simple, and Wrong

There seems to be one piece of advice upon which virtually all nutritional authorities agree. Eating less salt will lower your blood pressure and therefore reduce the risk of heart disease. And people are listening: More than 50 percent of Americans try cutting back on salt with about 25 percent being advised by their health-care professional to do so. Americans eat approximately 1½ teaspoons of salt per day, but the recommended amount is less than half this quantity. This advice is clear, simple, and just plain wrong.

We have not always condemned salt as a dietary villain. As Dr. DiNicolantonio covers in his book, *The Salt Fix,* entire cities have risen and fallen from the salt trade. People fought wars over salt. Throughout most of human history, salt was a vital nutrient. The word *salary* derives from the Latin word for salt—*sal.* Biblical passages speak of "salt of the earth." A common English saying is that somebody is "worth their salt." This linguistic evidence points to salt being a prized and important commodity rather than something that should be limited and shunned. When did we start to fear our natural craving for salt?[1]

In the 1950s, Lewis K. Dahl, a researcher from Upton, New York, noticed that people who ate less salt had less hypertension (high blood pressure), a key risk factor for heart disease.[2] Based on the limited data he had collected, Dahl promoted the notion that too much salt was the primary cause of hypertension and cardiovascular disease.

Dahl began to look for supporting evidence using genetically engineered salt-sensitive rats in his lab. Feeding massive amounts of salt to these rats predictably caused high blood pressure. Drawing conclusions from this study is fairly ridiculous. Because these rats were genetically manipulated to develop high blood pressure with salt, the results of this study were not proof of anything. The equivalent amount a human would need to consume is 4½ cups of salt per day, which is an outrageous amount! But Dahl extrapolated inappropriately to normal human babies and suggested that a high salt intake might contribute to early childhood mortality.[3] He was so influential with his assertion that food manufacturers began reducing salt in baby formula.

Dahl conjectured that salt was mildly addictive, and our cravings were triggered by eating it.[4] In 1976, Meneely and Battarbee suggested that Americans consume the bare minimum of salt compatible with life—just 3 grams of salt per day.[1] This unproven idea carried over into the first Dietary Goals for the United States in 1977, thereby becoming enshrined in nutritional lore. However, this recommendation was based almost solely on the questionable data from the studies of the genetically altered rats, and no human evidence existed at that time.

But the horse was already out of the barn. The government, the guidelines, and the media had already convinced the American public that salt was bad for their health despite the lack of any scientific backing. Over and over "experts" repeated the refrain of "avoid too much sodium." Repetition achieved what common sense could not, and salt restriction was written into dietary gospel. The first systematic review of clinical trials testing low-salt diets on blood pressure would not be published for almost *fifteen years* after the low-salt dogma had been almost universally accepted. Evidence would later suggest that our health woes were caused by another white crystal: sugar.[5]

By 1982, salt had been called "A New Villain" on the cover of *Time* magazine. The 1988 publication of the INTERSALT study seemed to seal the deal. This massive study laboriously measured salt intake and blood pressure in fifty-two centers across thirty-two countries. Sure enough, the higher the salt consumption, the higher the blood pressure. The idea that reducing dietary salt helped lower blood pressure seemed like a slam dunk, although the effect was quite small. A 59 percent reduction in sodium intake lowered the blood pressure by only 2 mmHg. For example, if your starting systolic blood pressure was 140 mmHg, then severe salt restriction could lower that to 138 mmHg. That's nothing to boast about. Further, no data existed as to whether this lower blood pressure would translate into fewer heart attacks and strokes. But based on this influential study, in 1994 the mandatory Nutrition Facts Label proclaimed that Americans should eat only 2,400 milligrams per day (about one teaspoon of salt).[6] Yet the stubborn fact remained that virtually every healthy population in the world eats salt at levels far greater than that recommendation. The dramatic improvements in health and life span of the last 50 years have occurred during a period where almost everybody was considered to be eating too much salt.

We largely base our belief in the benefits of low-salt consumption on misinformation and myth-information. We assume that too much salt is a recent phenomenon brought on by the increased consumption of processed foods. Dahl, for example, claimed in his writings that widespread use of salt as a condiment was uncommon until modern times, but we need only to study a little bit of history to see that this assertion was false.

Data from military archives from the War of 1812 show that soldiers (and presumably the rest of Western society) ate between 16 and 20 grams of salt per day.[7] Soldiers were given a daily salt ration of 18 grams per day despite its high cost to the army. American prisoners of war complained bitterly that their 9 grams per day of salt was "scanty and meager." It was only after World War II, when refrigeration replaced salting as the primary means of preserving food, that Americans lowered their average salt intake to 9 grams per day, where it has remained since. During the century before WWII, there was no concern of excess deaths from heart disease, stroke, or kidney disease—the main threats used to scare us into lowering our salt intake.

THE TIDES TURN

From the very beginning, it should have been obvious that lowering salt could not save lives. There were innumerable high-salt-eating cultures that had no adverse health consequences. The Samburu warriors[8] consume close to 2 teaspoons of salt per day, even going as far as eating salt directly from the salt licks meant for their cattle. Despite eating all this salt, their average blood pressure is just 106/72 mmHg and does not rise with age. In comparison, about one-third of the adult population in America is hypertensive, with a blood pressure of at least 140/90 mmHg or higher, despite the effort of trying to comply with dietary guidelines to reduce salt. For reference, normal blood pressure is less than 120/80 mmHg and generally rises with age in the United States. Villagers from Kotyang, Nepal eat *2 teaspoons of salt per day*, and the Kuna Indians eat *1½ teaspoons of salt per day*, with no hypertension.[9] The chart in Figure 10.1[10] shows many other examples that contradict Dahl's hypothesis that a high-salt diet causes hypertension.

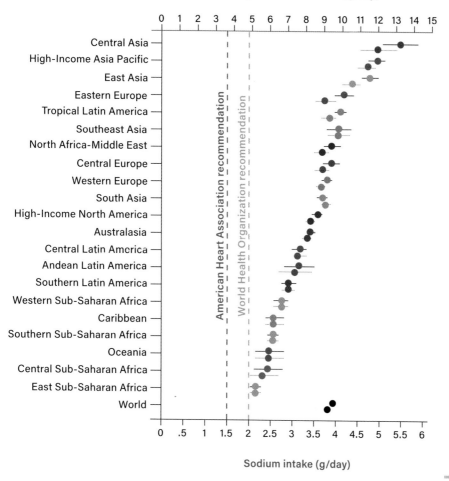

Fig. 10.1

The most recent survey of global salt intake from 2013 shows that no area of the world conformed to either the American Heart Association (AHA) or the World Health Organization (WHO) recommendations for salt restriction. The central Asian region had the highest salt intake, followed closely by the Asia Pacific region including Japan and Singapore. The Japanese diet is notoriously high in sodium because of the soy sauce, miso, and pickled vegetables they eat. The Japanese seem to suffer no ill effect and have the world's longest life expectancy at 83.7 years. Singapore is third in life expectancy at 83.1 years. If eating salt was so bad for health, how could the world's longest-lived people also eat one of the world's saltiest diets?

Scientific concerns about the validity of the low salt advice started in 1973 when an analysis[11] found six populations where the average blood pressure was low despite an extremely high-salt diet. For example, those living in Okayama, Japan, consumed more salt than most nations today (up to 3⅓ teaspoons per day), and yet had some of the lowest average blood pressures in the world.

In some cases, blood pressure *decreased* as salt intake increased. For example, North Indians consumed an average salt intake of 2½ teaspoons (14 grams) per day but maintained a normal blood pressure of 133/81 mmHg. In South India, average salt intake was about half that of North India, but the average blood pressure was significantly higher at 141/88 mmHg.[12] If salt was truly one of the major determinants of blood pressure, then this anomaly should not exist.

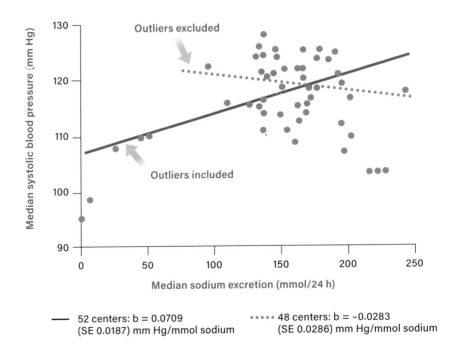

Fig. 10.2: INTERSALT: higher salt intake, lower blood pressure[13]

— 52 centers: b = 0.0709
(SE 0.0187) mm Hg/mmol sodium

••••• 48 centers: b = −0.0283
(SE 0.0286) mm Hg/mmol sodium

But there was still the question of the massive INTERSALT study, which people often cite as the ultimate proof of the harm of eating too much salt (see Figure 10.2). Further analysis of the data began to paint a significantly different picture. Researchers included four primitive populations (the Yanomamo, Xingu, Papua New Guinean, and Kenyan) in the initial analysis, and those societies had significantly lower sodium intakes than the rest of the world. (One had a sodium intake 99 percent lower!) However, they also lived a vastly different, primitive lifestyle from the others. These outliers had limited generalizability to the rest of the world, and, because they were such outliers, they had an outsized effect on the averages.

These four primitive societies differed from modern ones in far more than just diet. For example, the Yanomami Indians of Brazil still live traditionally, hunting and gathering just as they had done centuries ago. They practice endocannibalism (in which people consume the ashes of loved ones) because they believe it keeps them alive. They don't eat processed foods (because they don't have any). They don't use pesticides or preservatives. They don't use modern medicine. Comparing a Yanomami Indian living in the jungles of the Amazon to a person living in the jungles of New York is hardly fair. Isolating a single component of their diet (sodium) and proclaiming it to be solely responsible for high blood pressure is the pinnacle of bad research. You could just as easily conclude that wearing loincloths and eating the ashes of your dead relatives lowers your blood pressure.

There were other concerns with the INTERSALT study, too. Two populations (Yanomami and Xingu Indians), when studied further, had the near absence of a specific gene D/D of the angiotensin-converting enzyme (ACE), which put these populations at extremely low risk of heart disease and hypertension regardless of how much salt they ate. Thus, low sodium intake may not be the major or even minor contributor to low blood pressure in these groups. Rather, these two populations may have low blood pressure for genetic rather than dietary reasons.

In cases where there are significant outliers, the proper scientific analysis would be to analyze the information by removing these outliers to see if the original salt hypothesis still holds. When those four primitive populations were removed, and the remaining forty-eight Westernized populations were analyzed, the results were opposite the original findings. *Blood pressure decreased as salt intake increased.* Eating less salt was not a healthy practice; it was harmful. We shouldn't be eating less salt. We should be eating *more*. This study would not be the only one to confirm these surprising results.

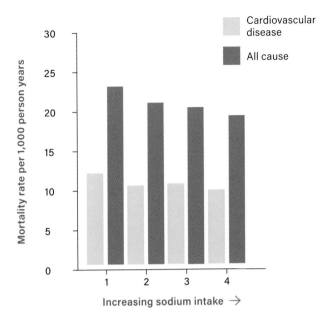

Fig. 10.3: NHANES I: Higher salt intake, lower risk of death[14]

We have consistent evidence from American studies that shows that eating less salt is associated with poor health. The National Health and Nutrition Examination Survey (NHANES) is a periodic, large-scale survey of American dietary habits. The first survey[15] found that those people who ate the least salt died at a rate 18 percent *higher* than those who ate the most salt (see Figure 10.3). This finding was a highly significant and exceedingly disturbing result. Eating low-salt diets was not healthful but harmful. It also confirmed the problem of salt restriction seen in the INTERSALT study.

The second NHANES survey confirmed the horrible news that a low-salt diet was associated with a staggering 15.4 percent increased risk of death. Other trials found an increased risk of heart attacks of eating a low-salt diet in treated hypertensive patients. Those were precisely the patients to whom doctors had been recommending a low-salt diet! We weren't healers; we were killers.

In 2003, the Centers for Disease Control, part of the U.S. Department of Health and Human Services, became worried and asked the Institute of Medicine (IOM) to take a fresh look at the available evidence to focus on mortality and heart disease rather than the surrogate outcome of blood pressure.[16] In other words, the IOM took on the task of finding out if salt restriction could reduce heart attacks and death, which are outcomes that matter more than merely making a few blood pressure numbers temporarily look better.

After an exhaustive search of the medical literature, the IOM made several major conclusions. Although low-salt diets could lower blood pressure, "Existing evidence... does not support either a positive or negative effect of lowering sodium intake to less than 2,300 milligrams per day in terms of cardiovascular risk or mortality in the general population."[17] That is, eating less salt did not reduce the risk of heart attack or death. However, in patients with heart failure, "The committee concluded that there is sufficient evidence to suggest a negative effect of low sodium intakes." Oh my. In other words, in patients with heart failure, eating less salt was bad, very bad. One of the very first things that millions of doctors learned in medical school was to advise patients with heart failure to eat less salt. This was exactly wrong, and decidedly deadly, advice.

But dogma is hard to change. Sticking our heads in the sand is easier than admitting we were wrong. Ignoring the advice of the IOM, the 2015 Dietary Guidelines continued to recommend reducing sodium intake to less than 2,300 milligrams of sodium (about one teaspoon of salt) per day, whereas the American Heart Association recommends less than 1,500 milligrams of sodium per day.

WHY IS SALT RESTRICTION DANGEROUS?

Salt is crucial for maintaining an adequate blood volume and blood pressure to ensure that our tissues are perfused with oxygen-carrying blood and nutrients. Salt is composed of equal parts sodium and chloride. When we measure the electrolytes in the blood, sodium and chloride (salt) are by far and away the most common ions. For example, normal blood contains sodium at a concentration of approximately 140 mmol/L and chloride at 100 mmol/L. Potassium concentration in the blood is only at 4 mmol/L, and calcium is at 2.2 mmol/L. There is more than 50 times more sodium than calcium in the blood. No wonder we need salt so badly.

There is speculation about the evolutionary reasons why our blood evolved to be mostly salt. Some believe that we evolved from single-celled organisms in Earth's ancient seas. As we developed multicellularity and moved onto land, we needed to carry some of the ocean with us as "salt water" inside our veins; hence, salt comprises the vast majority of the electrolytes of the blood. Salt is vital, not a villain.

The unintended consequences of the low-salt advice have been conveniently swept under the rug. For example, eating less than ½ teaspoon of salt per day can lower blood volume by 10 to 15 percent.[18] This may lead to low blood pressure upon standing (orthostatic hypotension), cause dizziness, and, potentially, result in a bone-breaking fall. Low-salt intake increases erectile dysfunction, sleep disturbances, and fatigue.[19]

During exercise,[20] the average person sweats more than two-thirds of a teaspoon of salt per hour.[21] That's the amount the AHA suggests you take for the entire day! With limited reserves of salt in the body, you can quickly develop low blood volume and dehydration.

Salt also makes food taste sweeter, so less salt on your food may mean that you end up eating more sugar as a way to compensate. In fact, salt has been blamed for many of the ills that are caused by sugar, including hypertension, chronic kidney disease, and cardiovascular disease.[22] We blamed the wrong white crystal.

Experts recommended salt restriction because they believed that less salt in the diet could decrease blood pressure without any harmful side effects. However, this assumption has long been known to be incorrect. As early as 1973, an editorial in the prestigious *New England Journal of Medicine* worried that when salt is restricted, the hormones aldosterone, angiotensin II, and sympathetic tone increase. High levels of all these hormones are known to be bad for heart disease, which is the very reason we block them with lifesaving medications such as spironolactone, ACE inhibitors, and beta-blockers. Thus, doing something that might raise these hormones, such as restricting salt, is potentially dangerous or, even lethal. This increased risk was borne out in a 2011 study.[23] Those patients who ate the least salt had more than three times the rate of cardiovascular death compared to those who ate the most. Eating a low-salt diet was bad, very bad (see Figure 10.4).

What's more, a low salt intake has been consistently found to worsen insulin resistance[24] and increase fasting insulin levels,[25] which potentially increases fat gain because insulin is a fat-storing hormone. Thus, the low-salt advice might increase your risk of developing diabetes and obesity. Along with raising artery-stiffening hormones,[26] the low-salt advice causes the very diseases

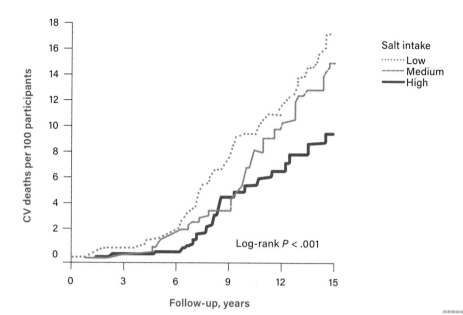

All cardiovascular disease events

Salt intake
········ Low
------- Medium
—— High

Log-rank *P* < .001

CV deaths per 100 participants

Follow-up, years

it supposedly prevents: hypertension, kidney disease, heart failure, and cardiovascular disease. What delicious irony.

These findings explain why countries that eat a salt-heavy diet—like Japan, South Korea, and France—also have some of the lowest rates of coronary heart disease mortality in the world and live the longest.[27] The most recent, largest, and most rigorous population study ever done—Prospective Urban Rural Epidemiology (PURE)—confirmed what we should already have known. The study examined more than 100,000 people in seventeen countries, and the data conclusively found that the lowest risk of death for cardiovascular events was in those people who consume between 3,000 and 6,000 milligrams of sodium per day.[28] Conveniently, Americans average 3,400 milligrams of sodium intake daily, which is right in the sweet spot. Another meta-analysis in almost 275,000 patients came to virtually the same conclusion. Consuming between 2,645 to 4,945 milligrams of sodium per day was associated with the lowest risk of death and cardiovascular events.[29] So the best current evidence suggests that the optimal intake of sodium is between 3,000 and 6,000 milligrams per day which is in direct contrast to sodium restriction recommendations of 2,300 milligrams of sodium or less.

THE PREMATURE CONVICTION OF SALT AS A DIETARY VILLAIN

We need salt to live, so our bodies tightly regulate the salt level in our blood. If we couldn't do this, we would all be dead. When we become salt depleted, we crave it.[30] For you, this may manifest as absentmindedly reaching for popcorn or potato chips, but your hunger for salt has evolved over 100 million years,[31] and it has helped all land animals, including humans, to survive. During salt depletion, our kidneys hold onto the precious salt like Ebenezer Scrooge holds onto his precious pennies. When we eat too much salt, the kidneys simply pass it out through the urine.

Our brain automatically and unconsciously controls our salt craving,[32] just as it controls our thirst for water. You don't manage your salt levels by adjusting your diet; your body maintains a steady salt level regardless of how much or how little salt you eat. The amount of salt in your body, which is so critical to your overall well-being, is not left up to the vagaries of what you put in your mouth, which changes from hour to hour, day to day, and season to season.

An overturn of the premature conviction on salt should have occurred with the publication of a 2014 Cochrane meta-analysis,[33] which found that a salt-restricted diet minimally reduced blood pressure, but there were no significant reductions in death or cardiovascular disease. A 2016 systemic analysis concluded once again that low-salt diets did not lower blood pressure in patients without hypertension.[34] Millions of people with normal blood pressure who try to eat less salt get no benefit from their efforts. So, why recommend salt restriction for the entire population of the world? How much more evidence do we need to overturn the low-salt advice?

If you still fear the salt shaker, know that your fear is not based on fact. Don't feel guilty about salting your food and recognize that salt is an essential micronutrient. To this day, there is still no definitive proof that restricting our salt intake will improve health, but there is strong evidence that consuming a normal salt intake will prolong life and reduce strokes and heart attacks. For years we have gotten it wrong about salt, and our health has been suffering for it ever since. We need to bring salt back to its cherished place at the dinner table.

OBTAIN A QUALITY SALT

Because of pollution, sea salts can be contaminated with plastics and heavy metals, so choose a salt that comes from an underground ancient ocean, such as Redmond Real Salt (www.realsalt.com), which has the additional advantage of a high iodine concentration. Most sea salt contains little to no iodine, but it often includes artificial potassium *iodide* that the manufacturer adds. Redmond Real Salt *naturally* contains *iodine* and therefore does not require iodide. Getting sufficient iodine is important because you can lose anywhere from 50 to 100 micrograms of iodine in sweat per hour of exercise in the heat. If you are constantly exercising and sweating out iodine but not replacing, the result could be hypothyroidism, weight gain, and metabolic issues. Give yourself a Salt Fix, throw out that processed table salt and pick up a healthy unrefined salt like Redmond Real Salt.

We need to bring salt back to its cherished place at the dinner table.

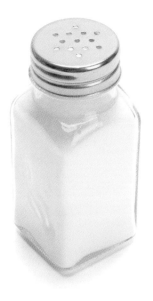

Magnesium: The Other Salt

Magnesium is one of the most common ions in the human body. The human body contains around 25 grams of it, with 99 percent of it inside the cell and just 1 percent of it in the blood. Magnesium is necessary for the proper functioning of at least 600 enzymes[35]— including the important Na-K-ATPase, DNA, and RNA—and protein synthesis.[36] The elimination of magnesium from your body is mainly controlled by the kidneys.

The Recommended Daily Allowance (RDA) for magnesium is 420 milligrams per day for men and 310 to 320 milligrams per day for women. Excess heavy metals, the use of fertilizers and pesticides, and soil erosion have dramatically reduced the amount of magnesium in our food supply.[37] Additionally, refined carbohydrates have virtually no magnesium because the manufacturing process of the foods has eliminated it.[38] Consequently, an estimated 50 percent of Americans consume less than the RDA, and some age groups consume substantially less than 50 percent.[39] The average intake of magnesium in the United States has been estimated at just 228 milligrams per day in women and 266 milligrams per day in men.[40] The amount of magnesium needed to maintain positive balance sits somewhere between 180 and 320 milligrams of magnesium for most people.[41] Thus, many Americans may be slowly depleting the magnesium from their muscles, bones, and organs every day. Subclinical magnesium deficiency is present in up to 30 percent of the American population.[42]

There are more than sixty factors that cause magnesium deficiency.[43] Some of the most common include consuming and using alcohol, sugar, antacids (and other stomach-acid-suppressing therapies), calcium supplements, and diuretics; gastrointestinal disorders (celiac disease, Crohn's, and ulcerative colitis); vitamin D excess or deficiency; and sodium deficiency. Magnesium deficiency is very hard to diagnose because symptoms are nonspecific, and blood magnesium levels may be normal even when there's an overall deficiency. Less severe signs of magnesium deficiency include anxiety, muscle cramps, disorientation, involuntary muscle contractions, muscular weakness, photosensitivity, spasticity, tinnitus, and tremors. The more severe signs of magnesium deficiency include arrhythmias, calcifications of soft tissue, cataracts, convulsions, coronary artery disease, depression, hearing loss, heart failure, hypertension, migraines, headaches, mitral valve prolapse, osteoporosis, seizures, and sudden cardiac death.

Magnesium deficiency causes an accumulation of calcium within the cell, leading to calcification of the arteries, which is sometimes called *hardening of the arteries*. Think of magnesium as a natural calcium blocker because it prevents calcium from accumulating where it shouldn't. Magnesium deficiency also increases oxidative stress and lipid peroxidation in the body and leads to coronary artery spasms that can be fatal.[44] Ensuring adequate dietary magnesium intake has been associated with lower risks for hypertension, arrhythmias, calcifications, heart failure, myocardial infarction, stroke, and sudden death.[45]

Many people following a low-carb, high-fat diet might not be getting enough magnesium. Dietary fat can reduce the absorption of magnesium,[46] and many good dietary sources of magnesium, such as dark chocolate, beans, nuts, seeds, bananas, and unrefined whole grains, are relatively scarce in a low-carb, high-fat diet. Following a higher protein diet also increases the need for magnesium. Thus, eating more protein or more fat increases the need for magnesium, but foods higher in protein or fat tend to also be relatively low in magnesium. If you follow one of these diets, you need to be aware of meeting your body's need for magnesium.

SALT AND MAGNESIUM: A CONNECTION LONG FORGOTTEN

Salt deficiency actually increases the risk for magnesium and calcium deficiency[47] and all the harmful consequences that come with it, such as hypertension, cardiovascular disease, heart failure, and kidney disease. Not so coincidentally, these are the very diseases we pin on consuming too much salt.

With a low-salt diet, the body pulls sodium out of the bones to maintain normal blood levels.[48] Unfortunately, the calcium and magnesium contained in bones are also stripped out, leading to deficiency. Low-salt diets may mean more magnesium lost in your sweat. When you restrict your salt intake, your body also increases the excretion of magnesium in sweat as a way to conserve sodium.[49] Additionally, the salt-retaining hormone, called aldosterone, skyrockets in the blood, which increases the excretion of magnesium through the urine.[50] The chance of magnesium being stripped from bones, excreted through sweat, and eliminated through urine poses a triple magnesium-depleting threat!

IS MAGNESIUM DEFICIENCY COMMON?

Magnesium deficiency affects at least 20 to 30 percent of the general population[51] and can cause heart arrhythmias, muscle spasms, and muscle cramps.[52] Magnesium deficiency is common and a serious public health problem, and it can lead to potassium and calcium deficiency. You can lose calcium because magnesium is required to activate vitamin D; when you're magnesium-deficient, that activation doesn't occur, and calcium deficiency results. On the flip side, magnesium deficiency increases the calcifications of arteries and blood vessels throughout the body. Salt depletion depletes the body of other healthy minerals such as magnesium, calcium, and potassium. In other words, you should consider sodium to be the "master controller" when it comes to the minerals in your body because it controls your magnesium status, which controls potassium and calcium.

Magnesium deficiency also can lead to increases in sodium and calcium within our cells, which may cause high blood pressure.[53] That's right, low-salt diets might *cause* high blood pressure by inducing magnesium (but also calcium and potassium) deficiency.

SUPPLEMENTAL MAGNESIUM

Most people need an additional 300 milligrams of magnesium per day (on top of what they're already getting in their diet) to lower their risk of developing numerous chronic diseases. So even if your average intake of magnesium is somewhere between 250 and 300 milligrams per day, an optimal intake might be around 500 to 600 milligrams of magnesium per day for most people, and it's perhaps even higher (up to 1,800 milligrams) for people with certain health conditions, such as hypertension or diabetes.[54]

Most magnesium supplements are the less expensive magnesium oxide form, which is not the best type. For the general population, magnesium glycinate (or diglycinate) has better absorption.[55] Adding vitamin B6 to magnesium supplements can increase its absorption and penetration into the cell.[56] Magnesium L-aspartate and magnesium chloride are also great choices with the greatest bioavailability of twenty different magnesium salts that have been tested.[57]

For those people suffering from kidney stones, magnesium citrate may be the best form to use because citrate can help reduce the formation of calcium-containing kidney stones.[58] For those people with heart failure, magnesium orotate at 6,000 milligrams once daily for one month and then 3,000 milligrams once daily for maintenance significantly reduces mortality.[59] However, the best way to get magnesium is from whole foods. Great options to get your daily dose of magnesium include cacao paste, nibs, beans, or powder from a company like Organic Traditions (http://organictraditions.com).

Don't Follow Dogma; Follow Evidence

You've been told for decades to eat less salt. This recommendation is dangerously outdated advice. These long-standing nutritional dogmas fall flat under the withering light of evidence-based medicine. The salt–blood pressure connection was oversimplified, and you've been suffering the consequences.

For the sake of your magnesium levels, think twice before restricting your salt intake. Eating more salt might help prevent magnesium deficiency to potentially reduce the risk of high blood pressure and cardiovascular disease. It's time you stopped fearing the salt shaker and started embracing your salt hunger; your magnesium levels might depend on it.

11

HEALTHY AND UNHEALTHY FATS

As we look back over the last forty years, it's hard to understand how we could have been as gullible as we've been. We believed that fat—more specifically saturated fat, which is the fat found primarily in animal foods—increased cholesterol and caused heart disease. To make matters worse, we were led to believe that we needed to switch to "heart-healthy" vegetable oils, like cottonseed, corn, safflower, and soy oils. Recent evidence suggests we were making a deal with the devil when we made this switch. The industrially processed seed oils were much worse than fat from animal sources. It was all a terrible mistake that began with Crisco.[1]

The Rise of Seed Oils

Cotton plantations were established in the United States as early as 1736 to cultivate cotton for fabric. Before this, cotton was largely an ornamental plant. At first, most cotton was home-spun into garments, but the success of the crop meant that some could be exported to England. A modest 600 pounds of cotton was produced in 1784; by 1790, that amount grew to more than 200,000 pounds. When Eli Whitney invented the cotton gin in 1793, the amount of cotton produced increased to a staggering 40,000,000 pounds.

But cotton is two crops: the fiber and the seed. The by-product of every 100 pounds of fiber produced from cotton was 162 pounds of cotton seeds, which were largely useless. Farmers needed only 5 percent of this seed for planting. Farmers could use some seed for livestock feed, but the remainder was still a mountain of garbage. What could farmers do with this garbage? In most cases, they left it to rot or illegally dumped it into rivers. It was toxic waste.

Meanwhile, in the 1820s and 1830s, a growing population in the United States resulted in an increased demand for oil for cooking and lighting. A decreased supply of whale oil for lamps meant that prices rose steeply. Enterprising entrepreneurs tried to crush the worthless cotton seeds to extract the oil, but it was not until the 1850s that the technology matured to the point that commercial production could commence. Then in 1859 something happened that would transform the modern world. Edwin Drake, who was known as Colonel Drake, struck oil in Pennsylvania and introduced a massive supply of fossil fuels to the market. Before long, the demand for cottonseed oil for lighting had completely evaporated, and cottonseeds were, once again, toxic waste.

Now cottonseed processors had lots of cottonseed oil on hand, but no demand. One solution was to add it illicitly to animal fats and lards. There was no evidence that this was in any way safe for human consumption. (We don't eat our cotton T-shirts, after all.) Cottonseed oil, which is light in flavor and slightly yellow, also was blended with olive oil to reduce costs. Italy, aghast at this crime against their culinary traditions, banned adulterated American olive oil in 1883. The Procter & Gamble company used cottonseed oil to manufacture candles and soap, but the company soon discovered that they could use a chemical process to partially hydrogenate cottonseed oil into a solid fat that resembled lard. This process produced what we now call trans fats. The hydrogenation made this product extremely versatile in the kitchen and gave it a longer shelf life, although nobody knew that they were putting something into their mouths that was formerly considered toxic waste.

This new solid vegetable oil made pastries, such as pie crusts, flakier. Because the hydrogenation gave the oil a longer shelf life, it could sit on a grocery store shelf for months without going rancid. It was smooth and creamy and as useful as animal fats in cooking for a fraction of the cost. Was it healthy? Nobody knew, and nobody cared. This new-fangled semisolid fat resembled food, so the manufacturer marketed it as food. The company called this revolutionary new Franken-product Crisco, which stood for *crystallized cottonseed oil.*

Crisco was skillfully marketed as a less expensive alternative to lard. In 1911, Procter & Gamble launched a brilliant campaign to put Crisco into every American household. They produced a recipe book (and all the recipes used Crisco, of course) and gave it away. This type of marketing campaign was unheard of at the time. Advertisements of that era also proclaimed that Crisco was easier to digest, cheaper, and healthier than lard because it was produced from plants. The ads neglected to mention that cottonseeds were essentially garbage. Over the next three decades, Crisco and other cottonseed oils dominated the kitchens of America, displacing lard.

By the 1950s, cottonseed oil was becoming expensive, so Procter & Gamble again turned to a cheaper alternative, soybean oil. The soybean had taken an improbable route to the American kitchen. Originally from Asia, where they had been domesticated in China as far back as 7000 BC, soybeans were introduced to North America in 1765. Soybeans are approximately 18 percent oil and 38 percent protein, which makes them ideal as food for livestock or industrial purposes (such as paint and engine lubricants).

Americans ate almost no tofu before World War II, so few soybeans made it into the American diet. Things began to change during the Great Depression when large areas of the United States were affected by severe drought. Farmers discovered that soybeans could help regenerate the soil through their ability to fix the nitrogen levels of the soil. It turns out that the great American Plains were ideal for growing soybeans, so they quickly became the second most lucrative crop, just behind corn.

Meanwhile, in 1924, the American Heart Association (AHA) was formed. At its inception, the AHA was not the powerful behemoth it is today; it was just a collection of heart specialists who occasionally met to discuss professional matters. In 1948, this sleepy group of cardiologists was transformed by a $1.7 million donation from Procter & Gamble (maker of hydrogenated trans fat–laden Crisco), and the war to replace animal fats with vegetable oils was on.

By the 1960s and 1970s, in a charge led by Ancel Keys, experts proclaimed the new dietary villain to be saturated fats, the type found most frequently in animal foods like meat and dairy. The AHA wrote the world's first official dietary recommendations in 1961 recommending that people "reduce [the] intake of total fat, saturated fat and cholesterol [and] increase [the] intake of polyunsaturated fat." In other words, people were encouraged to avoid animal fat and eat "heart-healthy" vegetable oils, which were high in polyunsaturated fats, like Crisco. This advice carried forward and was integrated into the influential 1977 Dietary Guidelines for Americans.

The AHA threw its now considerable influence into making sure that Americans ate less animal fat and less saturated fat. The Center for Science in the Public Interest (CSPI), for example, declared the switch from beef tallow and other saturated fats to trans-fat-laden partially hydrogenated oils "a great boon to Americans' arteries."[2] Don't eat butter, they said. Instead, replace it with the partially hydrogenated vegetable oil (read: trans fats) known as margarine. According to the CSPI, that edible tub of plastic was much healthier than the butter that humans had been consuming for at least 3,000 years, they said. Even as late as 1990, as the mountain of evidence was piling up that trans fats were supremely dangerous, the CSPI refused to acknowledge the dangers of trans fats. The group's famous bottom line was, "Trans, shmans. You should eat less fat."[3] Hydrogenation has many benefits for food manufacturers, including low cost and increased shelf life, but improved human health is not one of them. Ironically, these trans fat–laden margarines that the CSPI was promoting in place of animal fats[4] are more harmful than the fats they replace.[5]

In 1994, the CSPI struck fear into moviegoers' hearts with a brilliant scare campaign. At that time, movie popcorn was popped in coconut oil, which was largely saturated fat. The CSPI declared that a medium-size bag of movie popcorn had more "fat than a breakfast of bacon and eggs, a Big Mac and fries and a steak dinner combined."[6] Movie popcorn sales plunged, and theaters raced to replace their coconut oil with partially hydrogenated vegetable oils. Yes, trans fats. Additionally, the war to rid the American public of animal fat spilled over to beef tallow, which was the secret ingredient of McDonald's french fries. The fear of "artery-clogging" saturated fat resulted in the switch to—you guessed it—partially hydrogenated vegetable oils.

But the story was not yet done. By the 1990s, the trans fats that the AHA and the CSPI told us were supposed to be so healthy for us were implicated as major risk factors for heart disease. New studies indicated that trans fats almost doubled the risk of heart disease for every 2 percent increase in trans fat calories.[7] By some estimates, trans fats from partially hydrogenated vegetable oils were responsible for 100,000 deaths in the United States.[8] Yes, *100,000 deaths*. The very "heart-healthy" foods the AHA recommended were giving us heart attacks. Oh, the irony. By 2015, the U.S. Food and Drug Administration (FDA) removed partially hydrogenated oils from the list of Generally Recognized as Safe human foods. Yes, the AHA had been telling us to eat poison *for decades*.

The very "heart-healthy" foods the AHA recommended were giving us heart attacks.

Industrial seed oils, such as cottonseed, are high in the omega-6 fat linoleic acid. Linoleic acid is called the parent omega-6 fat because other omega-6 fats, such as gamma linolenic acid (GLA) and arachidonic acid, are formed from it. During Paleolithic times (2.6 million years ago until 10,000 years ago), linoleic acid came from whole foods, such as eggs, nuts, and seeds; humans would not have gotten any omega-6 from industrial seed oils. However, Crisco introduced an isolated and adulterated type of linoleic acid into our diet—one that was cheap, convenient, and highly damaging to our arteries. Since 1911, linoleic acid consumption has dramatically increased, and the source is one that humans had never consumed before. These omega-6 seed oils are now ubiquitous in nearly all manufactured foods, shelves of plastic bottles of seed oils line grocery store aisles. Unfortunately, these chemically unstable oils are highly susceptible to oxidation by heat, light, and air, and the oils get exposure to all three during their processing. Thus, although linoleic acid that comes from whole foods might be beneficial, the adulterated linoleic acid found in industrial seed oils is not. For a deeper dive on this topic, check out Dr. DiNicolantonio's book *Superfuel: Ketogenic Keys to Unlock the Secrets of Good Fats, Bad Fats, and Great Health*.

So how do we know which are healthy fats and which are unhealthy fats? Unsurprisingly, natural fats, whether they come from animal (meat, dairy) or plant sources (olive, avocado, nut) are generally healthy. Highly processed, industrial seed oils and artificially hydrogenated trans fats are unhealthy. Let's face it; we ate vegetable oils because they were *cheap*, not because they were healthy. Let's dig in to more details.

Basic Facts on Fats

Dietary fats are generally divided into two types: saturated and unsaturated (which includes monounsaturated and polyunsaturated). A saturated fat is so named because its carbon "backbone" is saturated, or full with, hydrogen atoms, and it can't accept any more. A monounsaturated fat, such as the oleic acid in olive oil, has space to accept one extra hydrogen (*mono* means *one*), and polyunsaturated fats can accept many hydrogens (*poly* means *many*).

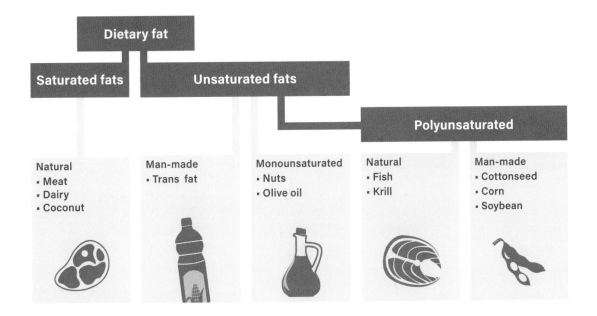

All natural sources of fat contain a mixture of all types of fat—saturated, monounsaturated, and polyunsaturated. However, the proportions vary. Animal sources, such as dairy or meat contain mainly saturated fats, whereas seed oils contain largely polyunsaturated fats of the omega-6 variety. Natural polyunsaturated fats, such as those in flaxseed and fatty fish, contain omega-3 fatty acids, including alpha-linolenic acid (ALA) (which is highly concentrated in flax) and docosahexaenoic acid (DHA) and eicosapentaenoic acid (EPA) (which are highly concentrated in seafood).

Although we tend to think of animal fats as saturated, bacon fat contains more oleic acid (a monounsaturated fat high in olive oil) than saturated fat. Chicken fat is approximately 50 percent monounsaturated compared to 30 percent saturated fat. Healthy olive oil contains almost 14 percent saturated fats. The highest concentrations of saturated fats are not in animal products but plant products; coconut oil is more than 90 percent saturated fat.

Fig. 11.1: The different types of fats

Fats to Avoid: Trans Fats and Industrial Seed Oils

What's shocking is that the very fats you've heard for decades are heart healthy (such as the trans fats and seed oils in Crisco) are the fats you want to avoid. In this section, we explain the harms of these fats, the studies, and the history of how you have been fed a big fat lie for more than a century.

INDUSTRIAL TRANS FATS

The recommendation to avoid trans fats is no longer controversial. The name derives from the alignment of the double bond found in many vegetable oils. The natural configuration of these fats is altered by artificial hydrogenation (adding hydrogen to unsaturated fats) that results in an unnatural configuration known as trans. Interestingly, natural trans fats found in ruminants such as sheep and goats do not appear to increase the risk of heart disease.[9]

Most nations of the world have either banned from use or are in the process of eliminating trans fats from their diet. In 2003, Denmark passed legislation that no more than 2 percent of fats and oils in any food product can contain trans fats.[10] As of June 18, 2018, the U.S. Food and Drug Administration ban on all trans fats from American restaurants and grocery store food items took effect. Canadians found their foods free of this Franken-fat by September 15, 2018. The World Health Organization issued a plan in 2018 to eliminate trans fats worldwide by 2023. Tom Frieden, a former head of the U.S. Centers for Disease Control said, "Trans fat is an unnecessary toxic chemical that kills, and there's no reason people around the world should continue to be exposed."[11]

VEGETABLE OILS

Vegetable oils, rich in omega-6, reduce cholesterol, so it was assumed that this reduction automatically translated into less heart disease. The human body can synthesize most of the different types of fats necessary for good health with two major exceptions—the essential fatty acids linoleic acid (an omega-6 fatty acid) and alpha-linolenic acid (an omega-3 fatty acid)—that we must obtain from the diet. Deficiency of either essential fatty acid results in disease. However, the ratio of omega-3 to omega-6 (see the table) is just as important because these two compete with each other for incorporation into human tissues and for the same rate-limiting enzymes.

The Omega-6-to-3 Ratio* of Common Oils

Dietary Source	Omega-6-to-3 Ratio
Grapeseed	696
Sesame	138
Safflower	78
Sunflower	68
Cottonseed	54
Corn	46
Peanut	32
Olive	13
Avocado	13
Soybean	7
Hemp seed	3
Chia seed	0.33
Flaxseed	0.27
Canola	0.2

* Table from *Superfuel* by Dr. James DiNicolantonio and Dr. Joseph Mercola. Copyright © 2018 by Dr. James DiNicolantonio and Dr. Joseph Mercola. Reprinted with permission of Hay House, Inc., Carlsbad, CA. The omega-6-to-3 ratio refers to LA/ALA.

It is estimated that an ancestral diet provided roughly equal amounts of omega-3 and omega-6 fatty acids. Plant omega-3 (ALA) is in foods like nuts, seeds, and beans, whereas marine omega-3 (EPA/DHA) is in seafood. Vegetable oils are almost purely omega-6. The dominance of industrial seed oils in the American diet has led to estimates that we consume ten to twenty-five times as much omega-6 as omega-3.

The AHA has long recommended replacing saturated fats with polyunsaturated fatty acids (PUFAs) like vegetable oil to reduce the risk of heart disease and death. However, recent trials have concluded that this is exactly wrong. When the advice originated in the 1960s, there was no distinction made between omega-3 and omega-6 fatty acids. Although both are PUFAs, their health effects are widely divergent. We have considerable evidence that the omega-3 fatty acids, such as DHA and EPA in fish oil, improve cardiovascular health. In contrast, overconsumption of the highly inflammatory omega-6 fatty acids in seed oils significantly worsen cardiovascular health.

The Sydney Diet Heart Study (SDHS) was a randomized controlled trial in which researchers replaced saturated fats with safflower oil, a concentrated source of omega-6.[13] This substitution was exactly the sort of thing the AHA had been advocating for years. Replace your butter with vegetable oil–based margarine. Those unfortunate enough to have followed this conventional advice in the SDHS suffered a 62 percent higher risk of death. The studies were showing that the "heart-healthy" seed oils were actually lethal.

The dangers of eating excessive omega-6 have long hidden behind some of the beneficial effects of omega-3. When the two fatty acids were analyzed separately, the dangers became obvious. In trials that included both omega-3 and omega-6, there was approximately a 20 percent reduction in death compared to saturated fat plus trans fat. However, trials that emphasized only omega-6, thereby raising the omega-6 to omega-3 ratio dangerously high, found a 33 percent *increase* in deaths, which was soon corroborated by other analyses (see Figure 11.2).[14]

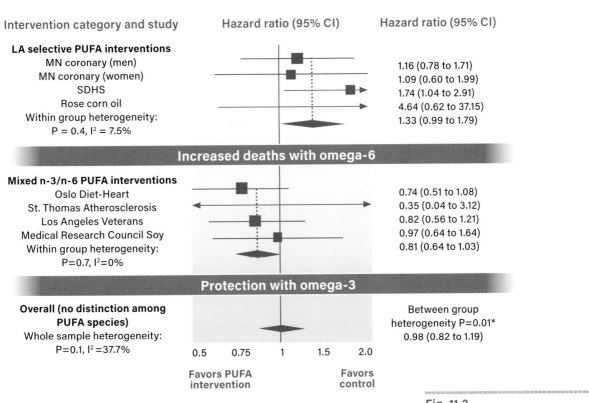

Intervention category and study	Hazard ratio (95% CI)	Hazard ratio (95% CI)
LA selective PUFA interventions		
MN coronary (men)		1.16 (0.78 to 1.71)
MN coronary (women)		1.09 (0.60 to 1.99)
SDHS		1.74 (1.04 to 2.91)
Rose corn oil		4.64 (0.62 to 37.15)
Within group heterogeneity: P = 0.4, I² = 7.5%		1.33 (0.99 to 1.79)

Increased deaths with omega-6

Mixed n-3/n-6 PUFA interventions		
Oslo Diet-Heart		0.74 (0.51 to 1.08)
St. Thomas Atherosclerosis		0.35 (0.04 to 3.12)
Los Angeles Veterans		0.82 (0.56 to 1.21)
Medical Research Council Soy		0.97 (0.64 to 1.64)
Within group heterogeneity: P=0.7, I²=0%		0.81 (0.64 to 1.03)

Protection with omega-3

Overall (no distinction among PUFA species)		Between group heterogeneity P=0.01*
Whole sample heterogeneity: P=0.1, I²=37.7%	0.5 0.75 1 1.5 2.0	0.98 (0.82 to 1.19)

Favors PUFA intervention   Favors control

Fig. 11.2

The harm from consuming industrial omega-6 seed oils might be due to an increase in oxidized linoleic acid metabolites (OXLAMs), which increase the susceptibility of LDL to oxidize, stimulate cancer, and lower HDL (high-density lipoproteins).[15] We recommend that you completely avoid consuming industrial seed oils. However, the moderate intake of linoleic acid from natural sources such as nuts, seeds, eggs, or chicken is safe because the linoleic acid from whole foods are protected from oxidation.

Unfortunately, the news would get much, much worse. The most rigorous study of changing our dietary fat from natural fats to industrial seed oils was done in the 1960s and 1970s. However, the results were suppressed and not fully available until 2016[16] after the original researcher had died, and other researchers retrieved the data from his son's basement to complete the analysis. In the study, the researchers replaced the natural saturated fats in the food with vegetable oils. The researchers compared findings for the test group to a separate group that was eating the usual diet.

This switch, of course, falls directly in line with the dietary advice the AHA has given for the past forty years without providing any proof that the substitution was beneficial. This study, which is known as the Minnesota Coronary Experiment, began with great promise as the vegetable oil group had lower blood cholesterols as expected. There was also a significant difference in mortality, but, in this case, the news was not good. Switching to vegetable oils increased the risk of death by a staggering 22 percent, and it was worse for patients older than 65. Making the switch isn't just bad; it's catastrophic.

The precise advice that governments around the world had been handing out to replace natural saturated fats with industrial seed oils high in omega-6 was exactly the opposite of what it should have been. We could hardly have done worse if we tried. Replacing natural foods like butter, cream, and meat that humans had been eating for millennia with industrially processed oil from garbage (cottonseed) is harmful. Vegetable oils were made to be cheap, not healthy.

Saturated Fats: PURE Study

It is somewhat counter-intuitive that saturated fats should have ever been considered more harmful than other fats. Unsaturated fats have multiple double bonds that enable them to accept other molecules, such as hydrogen. The result is that unsaturated fats are more chemically reactive than saturated fats that don't have these double bonds. When PUFAs like vegetable oil are left alone for too long, they become oxidized and rancid.

Saturated fats, like butter, are far less likely to suffer this problem, as they are more chemically stable. Hydrogenation can artificially change a PUFA into a saturated fat to create the Franken-fat nightmare of trans fats. We don't want our cells becoming rancid from the fats oxidizing inside our body, so if saturated fats are more stable, wouldn't consuming more saturated fat be good? The answer is yes.

In 2014, Dr. Dariush Mozaffarian, dean of Tufts University's Friedman School of Nutritional Science and Policy, did a thorough review of all available literature. He found that eating more saturated fats did not increase the risk of heart disease.[17] This finding closely echoes the findings from a 2010 analysis done by Dr. Ronald Krauss, director of atherosclerosis research at the Children's Hospital Oakland Research Institute, and Dr. Frank Hu from Harvard. Their analysis showed that eating more saturated fats was *not* associated with more heart disease, and paradoxically, it might be preventative for stroke.[18]

In 2017, Dr. Salim Yusuf performed the most comprehensive nutritional survey yet done: the Prospective Urban Rural Epidemiological (PURE) study. It spans eighteen countries and five continents; it followed more than 135,000 people for an average of 7.4 years. Given the overwhelming importance of diet and heart disease, it was vital to have rigorous evidence upon which to base national guidelines.

The PURE study showed eating more total or saturated fat *decreased* the risk of heart disease and death (see Figure 11.3).[19] Those subjects who ate the most fat had a 23 percent reduction in risk of death compared to those who ate the least fat, with similar results for saturated fat. The risk of heart disease was also 30 percent lower. The saturated fats that we had all feared as the cause of heart attacks were *protective*. The widely sanctioned and government-approved dietary guidelines to reduce total and saturated fats in our diets were completely divorced from reality. There was, and still is, no reason to avoid natural fats and saturated fats.

Eating a high-carbohydrate diet, as recommended originally in the 1977 Dietary Goals for the United States was also super harmful. In the PURE study, a high-carbohydrate diet was associated with a 28 percent increased risk of death and heart disease. Ironically, the advice for Americans to consume 55 to 60 percent of their calories from carbohydrates was the precise amount from this study that was the most lethal. The original USDA Food Pyramid made no distinction between processed and unprocessed carbohydrates, so the diet of Americans relied heavily upon the highly refined carbohydrates, like white bread and pasta, that were the most problematic.

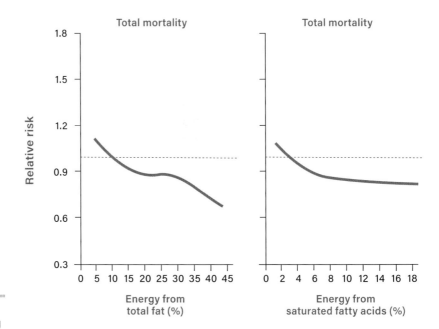

Fig. 11.3: Decreased mortality with increasing saturated fat intake

Good Fats: Monounsaturated

Replacing saturated with polyunsaturated fats was not good. But what about using monounsaturated fatty acids (MUFAs)? Most studies of MUFAs are problematic because of confounding by the variations in carbohydrate intake.[20] The Kanwu study shows that MUFA[21] improved insulin sensitivity in those taking a high-carbohydrate diet.

Switching patients from saturated fat (milk, butter, cheese, and fatty meat) to MUFA (olive oil, nuts, and avocados) resulted in slightly more weight loss, increased energy expenditure, and lower blood pressure despite equal caloric intake.[22] More importantly, the MUFA-rich diet improved the more dangerous fat around the abdomen—visceral fat. In other studies, the saturated fat palm oil raised insulin and lowered energy expenditure *when added to a diet high in sugar.*[23] The MUFA oleic acid, on the other hand, showed a slight *increase* in daily energy expenditure.[24]

Eating more monounsaturated fats might give you more wiggle room to eat more carbohydrates without becoming insulin resistant or gaining weight. Perhaps this is why many people living in the Mediterranean stay slim and healthy while enjoying bread and pasta. First, they enjoy these foods without *gorging* on them with bottomless bowls and multiple refills. Second, the high-carb foods often are accompanied by a generous drizzle of olive oil. A large analysis of fifty epidemiological and randomized controlled studies encompassing more than 500,000 people found that adherence to a Mediterranean diet can improve waist circumference, HDL, triglycerides, blood pressure, and blood glucose levels.[25]

Oleic acid (the predominant fat in olive oil) has a greater *oxidation rate* than stearic acid (a saturated fat found in beef and chocolate).[26] The result is that it liberates more energy, which increases satiety and reduces subsequent food intake. It also increases fat burning at the cellular level[27] and requires more energy for digestion.[28] These things are true even for obese post-menopausal women, a group that has a notoriously difficult time losing weight.[29] Switching from cream to olive oil allowed these women to use more fat for cellular energy rather than carbohydrate. If you want to *lose* body fat, you've got to use body fat, not carbohydrate.

Strategic fats for a higher carb diet include more nuts, olive oil, and avocados, and less fatty meat and full-fat dairy (cheese, milk, butter). If you do follow a low-carb diet and the occasional "cheat day" sneaks in, it might be better to try to get fats from monounsaturated sources than from saturated sources. (Skip the meat-lovers pizza and opt for sushi, with lots of avocado along with the rice.)

Natural saturated fats are fine, but for weight loss, consider replacing them with monounsaturated fat, especially if you favor a more moderate carb intake rather than a low-carb diet.

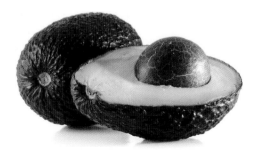

The Benefits of Consuming Less Saturated Fat and More Monounsaturated Fat

The following are some effects of consuming less saturated fat and more monounsaturated fat for those consuming a diet moderate to high in carbohydrates:[30]

- Greater weight loss and fat loss
- Less loss of muscle and lean tissue
- Reduced blood pressure
- Greater post-meal fat oxidation (burning fat rather than carbohydrate)
- Lower post-meal triglycerides
- Higher post-meal HDL

Medium-Chain Triglycerides and Coconut Oil

Coconut oil is rich in the medium-chain-length saturated fatty acids lauric acid and myristic acid. Most dietary fats are composed of carbon chains that have twelve to twenty-two carbons. Medium-chain triglycerides (MCTs) have only six to twelve carbons, and this shorter length might provide some health benefits. Coconut oil has MCTs; other sources might include palm kernel oil, butter, and whole milk.

The shorter chain length makes it possible for the body to absorb MCTs more rapidly, so they're quickly converted to ketones and metabolized for fuel. Technically speaking, MCTs are absorbed directly into the portal circulation that goes from the intestines to the liver. The lymphatic system absorbs longer-chain fatty acids into the blood; from there, the fatty acids go to the fat cells for storage, so much of it never makes it to the liver. In the liver, MCTs cross the mitochondrial membrane quickly (mitochondria are the power-producing parts of cells), and carnitine doesn't need to be present for this to happen. In short, MCTs go directly to the liver, where they are metabolized much more quickly into energy. This accelerated metabolic conversion into fuel means that potentially less is stored as body fat and more is burned for fuel.

Coconut oil does raise total cholesterol, but it preferentially increases HDL, the "good" cholesterol, which explains some of its reported heart benefits.[31] And "virgin" coconut oil, which is similar to virgin olive oil, is even healthier because it's extracted solely through mechanical means without heat or chemicals and retains all of the bioactive polyphenols typically lost in refinement.[32] Organic Traditions makes a great organic raw coconut oil.

Human studies using MCTs show some promising results, including greater weight loss compared to olive oil[33] and longer-chained saturated fats.[34] The greater weight loss may be attributable to appetite suppression or increased energy expenditure. Fast conversion of MCTs to energy activates satiety mechanisms to stop eating, which has huge significance in weight loss efforts. High MCT intake led to significantly lower overall calorie consumption—in one study, an average of 256 fewer calories per day,[35] and 41 to 169 calories per day in another study.[36]

MCT oil might increase energy expenditure when it's substituted for other oils.[37] Dr. Marie-Pierre St-Onge, an associate professor of nutrition at Cornell University Medical School who has been studying MCTs for almost two decades, says, "Coconut oil has a higher proportion of medium-chain triglycerides than most other fats or oils, and my research showed eating medium-chain triglycerides may increase the rate of metabolism more than eating long-chain triglycerides."[38] A diet with 30 grams of MCTs increased twenty-four-hour energy expenditure by 114 calories.[39] Although these overall effects are relatively small, the combination of increased energy expenditure with decreased appetite over long periods might hold significant benefits.

MCTs lack the polyphenols found in many foods high in MUFA (such as avocados, olives, and nuts). However, coconut oil significantly raises HDL. Traditional populations in the South Pacific that subsisted on large amounts of coconuts, loaded with coconut oil, maintained excellent health for generations. The traditional foods on the islands of Kitava, Trobriand Islands, and Papua New Guinea included roots, fish, and coconut. Studies of this diet found the "apparent absence of stroke and ischaemic heart disease."[40]

A high intake of the saturated fats in coconut oil did not "clog" arteries. Instead, there was virtually no heart disease at all.

The Tokelau migrant study demonstrates once again the potential benefits of coconut oil.[41] The small South Pacific island of Tokelau lies northeast of New Zealand, and for generations the locals subsisted on fish, breadfruit, and coconut. It was estimated that 70 percent of their calories were derived from coconut, so their diet was extremely high in saturated fat—almost 50 percent. Early descriptions of their health noted low levels of high blood pressure, heart disease, obesity, and diabetes. In 1966, a tropical cyclone forced the evacuation of a significant portion of the population to New Zealand. The emigration forced by the cyclone provided a unique opportunity to study the effects of changing to a typical Western diet, which was higher in sugar and refined carbohydrates and much lower in saturated fat. The news was not good.

In a comparison of the Tokelauan emigrants and those who stayed on the island, the average weight of male emigrants increased by twenty to thirty pounds over the ensuing decade. Diabetes more than doubled in the population. Blood pressure rose by an average of 7.2 mmHg systolic and 8.1 mmHg diastolic, and gout increased. Replacing the traditional diet heavy in coconut and coconut oil with a Western diet was hugely detrimental to the Tokelauans' health.

Full-Fat Dairy

For years, we've been told to eat low-fat dairy or drink skim milk with the assumption that the milk fat, which is highly saturated, was detrimental to our heart health. This assertion is a direct contradiction of the wisdom of the previous millennia during which dairy was prized specifically for its high fat content. In English, there are many phrases like:

- The cream always rises to the top.
- This is the cream of the crop.
- You're skimming off the top.

All of these sayings have the same connotation: The cream, the fattiest part of the milk, is also the most desirable.

With the heavy emphasis on eating low-fat dairy, you might think that many scientific studies had shown that dairy fat was unhealthy and that reducing milk fat was healthy. You might also be wrong. No evidence exists to prove that eating high-fat dairy causes heart disease.

Modern research exonerates dairy fat, this former villain.[42] A meticulous twenty-two-year follow-up of patients that measured blood markers of dairy fat found that eating dairy fat was not related in any way to the risk of heart disease or death. The study built upon a previous 2014 study that concluded there was no increased risk of stroke.[43] Lead author Dr. Marcia Otto pointed out that "the results suggest that one fatty acid present in dairy may lower risk of death from cardiovascular disease, particularly from stroke."[44] Yes, eating full-fat dairy was healthy, not harmful. A 2013 analysis suggests that dairy fat also might be protective against the development of type 2 diabetes, which is a growing epidemic worldwide.[45]

So, there is no longer a reason to be scared of eating full-fat dairy. Indeed, Dr. Arne Astrup, director of the Department of Nutrition at the University of Copenhagen, wrote in 2014 an article titled "A Changing View on Saturated Fatty Acids and Dairy: From Enemy to Friend."[46] This recent evidence shows why *Time* magazine proclaimed in 2016 that "butter is back."

Going Nuts

In the late 1990s, experts discouraged us from eating nuts largely because they are generally high in fat. Because all fats were considered bad, high-fat foods like nuts and avocados were also considered very unhealthy. But several large studies gradually pointed out the fact that eating nuts was associated with significant heart protection. This finding has now been replicated many times,[47] and the advice to eat more nuts is now widely accepted.

In this context, *nuts* include true tree nuts (almonds, hazelnuts, walnuts, and so on) and peanuts, which are a form of legume. Nuts contain primarily oleic acid, the same unsaturated fat found in olive oil, but they also contain plenty of fiber, protein, minerals, and polyphenols. Eating more nuts has been linked to a 13 percent reduced risk of type 2 diabetes, a lower risk of high blood pressure, and lower LDL cholesterol. These findings have prompted the AHA to recommend eating more nuts and seeds to reduce the risk of heart disease.[48] For each daily serving of nuts, studies estimate a reduction in risk of cardiovascular disease of 28 percent. Eating organic nuts, such as almonds, cashews, and hazelnuts, is an even better option. (Organic Traditions, which you can find at http://organictraditions.com, is a good source for organic nuts.)

Eating nuts was associated with significant heart protection.

Extra-Virgin Olive Oil: Going the "Extra" Mile

Extra-virgin olive oil (EVOO) and pure olive oil are both made from olives, but the two manufacturing processes are completely different. EVOO is an unrefined oil that's not treated with any chemical processes or heat. The oil is made by grinding olives into a paste and then cold-pressing them to extract the oil. EVOO is generally the highest-quality oil you can buy, and it has a price to match. The remaining paste still contains oil, so it can be treated with chemical solvents and heat to extract the remaining oil. This output becomes "pure" olive oil, which is generally cheaper than EVOO but is a refined oil that's of a lesser quality.

Extra-virgin olive oil is healthier than virgin olive oil because of its higher polyphenol content. A randomized, cross-over, controlled trial found that increasing the polyphenol content linearly increased the HDL and decreased the oxidized-LDL (the "bad" cholesterol). The authors of the study concluded, "Olive oil is more than a monounsaturated fat. Its phenolic content can also provide benefits

CHAPTER 11: Healthy and Unhealthy Fats

for plasma lipid levels and oxidative damage."[49] The phenolic compounds in EVOO have been noted to inhibit the oxidation of LDL, the process that makes LDL cholesterol so dangerous for the development of heart disease.[50] A study has shown that 50 grams of olive oil (just under 2 ounces) per day for just two weeks reduces LDL oxidation by 73 percent and macrophage uptake of LDL by 61 percent.[51] These numbers suggest that olive oil, especially EVOO, might reduce atherosclerosis.

Also, human studies show that EVOO lowers inflammation,[52] the "stickiness" of blood,[53] DNA damage,[54] oxidized LDL, and blood pressure, and it improves endothelial function.[55] For this reason, EVOO—especially a raw, ice-pressed organic olive oil such as Organic Traditions olive oil—is worth the extra mile for our health.

The Benefits of Marine Omega-3s

Consuming high amounts of marine omega-3s EPA and DHA has many health benefits, including fewer cardiovascular events and death.[56] Taking just 1 gram of EPA/DHA after a heart attack can reduce overall mortality, sudden cardiac death, and death. However, higher doses of EPA and DHA (3 to 4 grams per day) can reduce blood pressure, lower triglycerides, and stabilize atherosclerotic plaques.[57] Long-chain omega-3 fats reduce the risk for obesity by increasing basal metabolic rate and muscle protein synthesis while reducing muscle breakdown.[58] Fatty fish, such as salmon or sardines, are great sources of marine omega-3 fatty acids. However, there may be an even better source: krill oil.

Recommendations for EPA/DHA Supplementation

For maintenance of health and those with health conditions: We recommend consuming 3 to 4 grams of EPA/DHA per day from quality sourced wild seafood or a high-quality fish oil or algal oil supplement plus 3 to 4 grams of krill oil.

Krill Oil

Krill are tiny crustaceans (similar to shrimp) that live in the Arctic, Antarctic, and Pacific Oceans. Because krill are so small, they experience less heavy metal contamination than fish. The omega-3 fatty acids from krill provide enhanced absorption and penetration into the brain. A 1-gram dose of Neptune Krill Oil provides EPA/DHA (240 milligrams), vitamin A (100 IU), vitamin E (0.5 IU), phospholipids (400 milligrams), astaxanthin (1.5 milligrams), and choline (74 milligrams).[59]

Krill oil improves arthritis,[60] premenstrual syndrome, breast tenderness, and joint pain.[61] Krill oil at 1 to 3 grams per day is also more effective for reducing blood glucose, total cholesterol, and triglycerides and increasing HDL compared to fish oil and placebo.[62] Think of krill oil as "super omega-3" as it also contains astaxanthin, a highly potent antioxidant. Astaxanthin is unique because it can span across the entire lipid bilayer of the cell membrane and act as both a water- and fat-soluble antioxidant. Thus, astaxanthin prevents oxidative damage on the outside of the cell membrane and from the inside.

Prehistoric humans obtained "marine" omega-3s by consuming the brains of kills on the African Savannah.[63] Ounce for ounce, brain tissue is higher in DHA than salmon.[64] This source was more easily absorbed[65] and provided early humans with a unique "brain-DHA advantage." Eating brain is no longer routine, so supplementing with krill oil is the next best thing. Astaxanthin may help prevent the highly susceptible DHA in your brain from oxidizing, as it acts like a highly potent water- and lipid-soluble antioxidant.

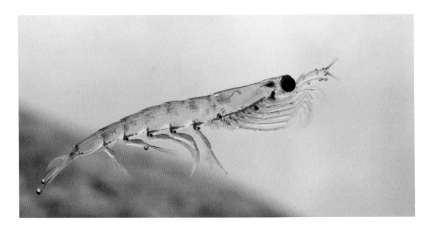

The Health Benefits of Krill Oil[66]

Krill oil is better absorbed and less likely to be oxidized than fish oil.

The omega-3s in krill are bound to phospholipids (which they aren't in fish oil). They can readily cross the blood-brain and blood-retinal barrier and deliver omega-3s into lipid bilayers to get to the sites that need them.

Krill oil provides phosphatidylcholine, which may help prevent fatty liver disease and improve cognition.

Astaxanthin penetrates skin cells to help prevent ultraviolet damage from sunlight.

Krill oil has greater antioxidant capabilities compared to fish oil.

It has an oxygen radical absorbance capacity (ORAC) value that is

   378 times greater than vitamin A and E

   47 times greater than fish oil

   34 times greater than CoQ10

   6.5 times greater than lycopene

Krill has a singlet oxygen quenching capacity that is

   6,000 times greater than vitamin C

   800 times greater than CoQ10

   550 times greater than vitamin E

   40 times greater than beta-carotene

Unlike fish oil, krill oil has no fishy burp or aftertaste.

It improves stiffness due to osteoarthritis.

Krill oil decreases

   C-reactive protein (CRP) by 30 percent

   Triglycerides by 28 percent

   LDL cholesterol up to 40 percent

It increases HDL cholesterol by 44 to 60 percent.

It significantly decreases fasting blood glucose levels by 6 percent.

Whereas fish oil decreased pericardial fat (fat around the heart) in rats by 6 percent, krill oil reduced it by 42 percent!

In rats, krill oil decreased liver fat by 60 percent, whereas fish oil decreased it only 38 percent.

Making Good Choices About Fats

The current classification of fats as saturated, monounsaturated (MUFA), or polyunsaturated (PUFA) is completely useless for understanding fats' effects on human health. This classification belongs in a chemistry book, not a book on health and longevity. Some fats are healthy (fats contained in whole foods), and some fats are unhealthy (industrially produced trans fats and vegetable oils). Saturated fats can be healthy, such as those found naturally in dairy and coconut oil. Polyunsaturated fats can be healthy (marine omega-3s) or unhealthy (industrial seed oils too high in omega-6 oils). More and more studies are finding the health benefits of monounsaturated fats found in olive oil, nuts, and meat. But artificial monounsaturated trans fats are extremely unhealthy. Knowing whether a fat is saturated or not does *not* help us understand whether we should eat them.

Instead, we can get a good idea of whether a fat is healthy by asking one simple question: Is it a natural fat? Those fats we find in nature, the ones we've been consuming as part of the human species for thousands of years, are not likely to be dangerous to our health. There are natural saturated fats (in dairy and coconut), natural monounsaturated fats (in olive oil), and natural polyunsaturated fats (omega-3 and omega-6). Research is now confirming the seemingly obvious notion that eating foods as close to their natural state as possible is healthy.

On the flip side are highly processed oils and fats. Trans fats are artificial unsaturated fats that we must avoid at all costs. This is almost universally understood. But avoiding highly processed, highly unnatural vegetable oils is just as important. Were our caveman ancestors opening a jar of sunflower oil to cook with? Or were they eating animal fat? It is the ultimate hubris to believe that humans can cook up an artificial, man-made fat such as vegetable oil that will be healthier than the fats that Mother Nature has made available for us to eat. Corn, for example, is not particularly oily. So, corn may be a natural food, but corn oil is not.

It's important to make sure that you consume healthy fats. These healthy fats, and foods that contain them, include extra-virgin olive oil, long-chain omega-3s, such as EPA and DHA, which are in seafood as well as fish, algal, and krill oil supplements, and the parent omega-3 fat, ALA, which is in flax and chia seeds. (Organic Traditions has a great variety of these seeds.) Even animal fats, such as butter, cheese, and milk seem harmless, especially when they come from pastured sources. You should avoid harmful fats, such as industrial trans fats and industrial omega-6 seed oils, at all costs.

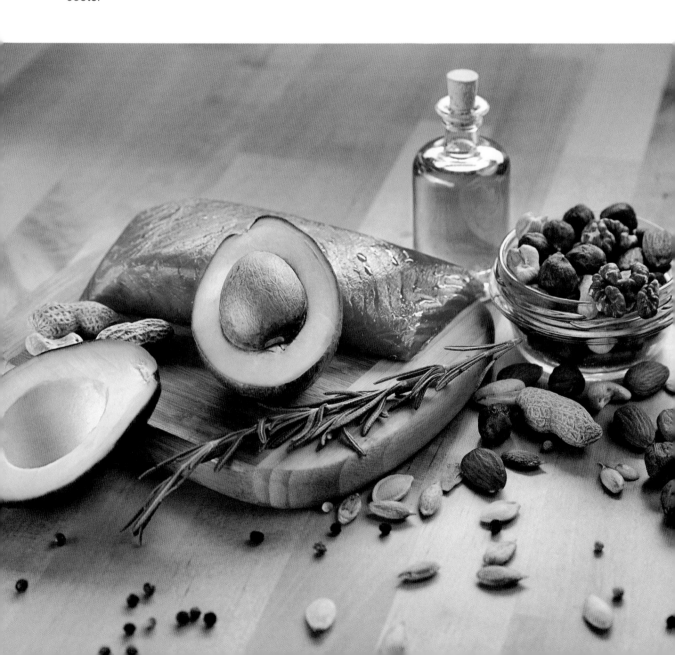

12

THE BLUE ZONES:

THE LONGEST–LIVING CULTURES

In 2005, *National Geographic* writer Dan Buettner used the term *Blue Zones* to describe certain areas of the world where people lived longer, healthier lives. The list of Blue Zones includes

- Okinawa, Japan

- Sardinia, Italy

- Loma Linda, California

- Nicoya Peninsula, Costa Rica

- Ikaria, Greece

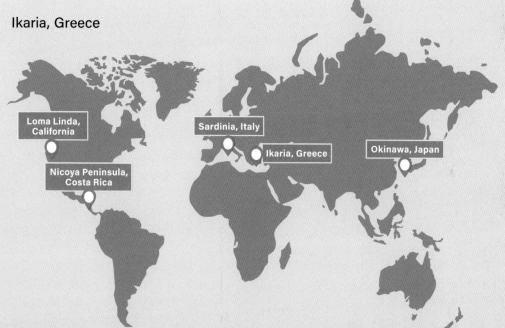

People living in these Blue Zone locations reach ages in their nineties, and even live past 100 (to become centenarians), with relatively little age-related disease. Although these people live throughout the world, with seemingly widely divergent diets and lifestyles, they all share certain characteristics that might help them live longer, fuller lives. These people often smoke less, move more (and at a moderate level), and prioritize family and socializing above all else. Their diet is often, but not always, plant-based, with relatively low protein intake, especially from animals. It is instructive to look a little more closely at the diets of these longevity superstars to learn their secrets.

Okinawa, Japan

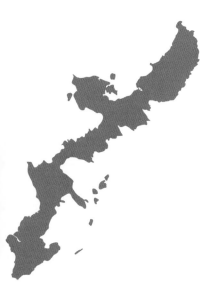

Across the world, the average number of people who live to be older than 100 is only 6.2 per 100,000. According to their 2017 census, Japan boasted the world's highest proportion of centenarians at 34.85 per 100,000. However, in 1990, the tiny Japanese prefecture of Okinawa crushed even that number with an astounding 39.5 per 100,000.[1] Okinawan men typically live to the age of 84, whereas the women live to an average age of 90 years, even though Okinawa is Japan's poorest prefecture and has the lowest number of physicians per capita. Citizens suffer small fractions of the rates of diseases that typically kill Westerners: 20 percent the rate of heart disease, breast cancer, and prostate cancer, and less than 50 percent the rate of Alzheimer's disease.[2] Tellingly, the diet in Okinawa has changed significantly in recent years to become more Westernized. By the year 2000, the Okinawan longevity advantage had largely vanished. Nevertheless, good data about the traditional diet of Okinawa can give us clues to their former longevity.

The traditional Okinawan diet contained some meat, particularly pork, along with plenty of plants. The oldest existing record of Japanese diets, which is from 1880, shows that Okinawans got an astounding 93 percent of their calories from the sweet potato.[3] They ate just under 40 grams of protein per day—a habit that persisted at least until 1949. Meals consisted of sweet potato, miso soup, and plenty of vegetables for breakfast, lunch, and dinner.

The traditional diet of Okinawans was about 80 percent carbohydrates, consisting of sweet potatoes, vegetables, and some grains. Just after World War II, Okinawans got nearly 70 percent of their calories from low-protein, nutrient- and fiber-dense sweet potatoes.[4] This diet is virtually the opposite of the Standard American Diet, which is low in nutrients (particularly potassium, magnesium, vitamin C, and carotenoids) and fiber.[5] Along with the ubiquitous sweet potato, other vegetables and legumes made up about 10 percent of the Okinawans' diet, and rice and other grains were responsible for nearly 20 percent. In 1988, the daily intake of pulses (beans) was 30 percent above Japan's national average, and the intake of green and yellow vegetables was 50 percent higher.

The Okinawan sweet potato ranges from red to deep yellow due to the high levels of anthocyanin. Both types of sweet potatoes are very high in polyphenols and antioxidants. Okinawa, which is a relatively isolated string of subtropical islands, has two growing seasons, which is favorable for the production of sweet potatoes and fresh vegetables. Rice grew poorly and was supplanted as the staple crop by the sweet potato in the 1600s.

Once a month, Okinawans held various festivals where they consumed meat, particularly fish and pork. Historically, meat and fish combined made up just a paltry 1 percent of calories, and dairy products and eggs were rare. The Okinawans' diet was nearly a vegan diet, and it supplied only about 1,800 calories a day[6] (compared to the 2,500 calories the average American consumes).

Over time, meat consumption increased. Residents of the coastal areas commonly ate fish; pork was the other common meat. Pigs were "free range," so they consumed wild plants, but people also fed them leftover vegetables rather than the grains farmers fed to pigs on feedlots in the West. Consequently, the meat from the free-range pigs was higher in omega-3 fatty acids and lower in omega-6 polyunsaturated fatty acids.

Sodium intake in the Okinawan diet is high, which is characteristic of all Japanese cuisine. The high levels of sodium come from the common use of soy sauce, miso, salted fish, and pickled vegetables.

One unique facet of Okinawan cuisine is the high consumption of the seaweed *kombu*. Although Japanese cuisine makes use of kombu for flavoring soups, the Okinawans eat large amounts of the seaweed directly. Kombu, which grows in seawater, is high in fiber, minerals, the marine omega-3 fats EPA and DHA, and salt; kombu contains a whopping 840 milligrams of sodium per ounce!

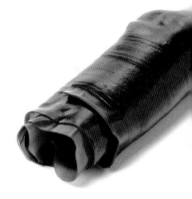

The low amount of protein was not detrimental to Okinawans' health or longevity. Their smaller stature and lower overall muscle mass mean we can't extrapolate this data to a muscular weight-lifting American, but it suggests that maybe we don't need as much protein as we once thought, especially if we're not doing intense resistance exercise.

Meat intake in Okinawa rose steadily in the post-World War II years, and by 1988, it had surpassed the Japanese average. Meat intake averaged 90 grams per person per day with an equal amount of pulses. Thus, the Okinawans did well with both a diet that was very low in protein and one that was relatively high in protein. Most Western cultures have a daily meat intake of more than 200 grams per day. (Note: A gram of meat is not the same as a gram of protein because meat might contain significant fat, depending upon the specific type of meat and cut.)

There were other changes in the modern Okinawan diet, too. The intake of pulses and green and yellow vegetables declined to the national average of Japan. The percent of calories from fat rose higher than 30 percent. The group of residents that have westernized their diet the most are younger residents, especially young men. They tend to avoid the traditional *champuru* dish, which contains meat (typically pork) or tofu that's stir-fried with vegetables. They also eat less fish than older generations.

Residents of Okinawa, like those in most parts of Japan and East Asia, drink copious amounts of tea. The most popular drinks are green tea and *kohencha*, a semi-fermented tea. In Okinawa, green tea is often scented with jasmine flowers and turmeric in a tea they call *shan-pien*, which loosely translates to *tea with a bit of scent*. The average Okinawan drinks at least 2 cups of tea daily.

The Okinawans traditionally follow an ancient Confucian tradition called *Hari Hachi Bu*. They stop eating before they are full; they only eat until they are *no longer hungry*. There's a profound difference between those two states. They deliberately stop eating when they are 80 percent full, a practice that has the same effect as a methodical 20 percent calorie reduction. To be able to stop eating before reaching fullness, Okinawans must practice what people often call *mindfulness eating*. If you are going to practice Hari Hachi Bu as the Okinawans do, you must constantly think about whether you are full.

You can follow some guidelines to make this deliberate calorie restriction easier:

- Remember that when you are eating, eat well.

- When you are not eating, *don't eat*. Never eat mindlessly. Don't eat in front of the TV. Don't eat and read. Don't eat in front of the computer. Concentrate upon what you are eating and enjoy it.

- When you are no longer hungry, stop eating.

- Eat slowly. Satiety signals in our stomachs take some time to register. If you eat until you are full, you can easily overshoot. Think about the last time you went to a buffet dinner. As you were eating, everything was fine. But after 10 or 15 minutes later, as all the satiety signals start to hit, you feel like you are going to explode. You might even be slightly nauseous.

- Use smaller plates or dishes to force yourself to get less food. We tend to eat everything on our plates because that habit has been ingrained into us since childhood. We clean our plates whether we have a lot of food or a little food. If we overfill our plates, we tend to keep eating until we finish everything, regardless of whether we are full. If we instead deliberately underfill our plates, then we can empty our plates without overeating, and we're forced to question whether we're still hungry before reaching for more food.

Unfortunately, the longevity advantage of Okinawans is quickly disappearing. After World War II, white bread and white rice started to replace the beloved sweet potato. Younger Okinawans are now eating more American-style fast food than ever, and many have become overweight. Intake of meat increased, and intake of green and yellow vegetables decreased. In fact, the obesity rate in the prefecture has become the highest in all of Japan.

It's likely that the traditional diet has played far more of a role in the Okinawans' long lives than anything in their lifestyle and environment.

Longevity Checklist: Okinawa

- ✓ **Calorie restriction/fasting:** Okinawans practice deliberate calorie restriction with Hari Hachi Bu.
- ✓ **mTOR:** The diets are low in animal protein.
- ✓ **Tea/coffee/wine:** Okinawans, like other Japanese, drink lots of tea.
- ✓ **Salt:** The meals are generally high in salt because of miso, kombu, and soy sauce.
- ✓ **Fat:** Fish is a staple of the diet, which is not high in fat, but low grains means a proper omega-6 to omega-3 ratio. No vegetable oils.

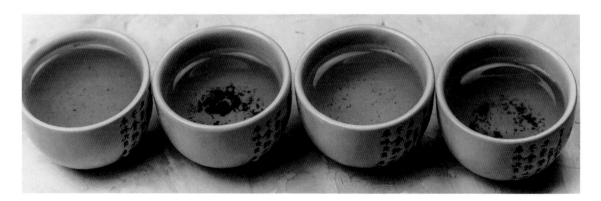

Sardinia, Italy

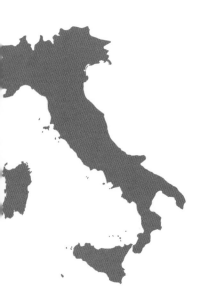

On the other side of the world from Okinawa is the Italian gem of Sardinia, which was the first Blue Zone to be identified. Sardinia lies in the Western Mediterranean basin 75 miles off the coast of Italy. Because of its mountainous terrain, residents have mostly lived in extreme isolation and relative poverty. Most of its centenarians reside in tiny villages dotted throughout the isolated inland of the island. At one point, one out of every 200 people in the small town of Ogliastra had made it past the century mark.[7] That's about fifty times the rate at which people in the United States reach 100 years old. Of further interest, the rate of centenarians has an unusually low female-to-male ratio of 2:1 rather than the typical 5:1 of other Blue Zones.[8] In Sardinia, the men were living past 100 years of age at a far greater rate than anywhere else in the world.

The first reliable accounts of the Sardinian diet come from French geographer Maurice Le Lannou, who described the diet as "remarkably frugal,"[9] which was likely due to the poverty of the region. One staple was vegetable soup (minestrone) that included copious amounts of fresh, locally grown vegetables. Cooks often added pulses to these soups, which people often ate with sourdough bread. Chestnuts and walnuts provided a substantial source of calories and monounsaturated fatty acids. Residents ate meat infrequently, as you might expect in an impoverished region. Reports from the mid-nineteenth century suggest that Sardinians ate meat only two to four times per month, although this rate has steadily increased over the years. Nevertheless, an estimated 70 to 83 percent of dietary protein came from vegetables even until the mid-twentieth century. Dairy consumption, however, was much higher than meat consumption, especially among the shepherds on the island. They mostly drank goat and sheep milk, and they ate ricotta cheese. Only people in the coastal regions ate fish.

The Sardinians, like their Italian cousins, drank a reasonable amount of wine, mostly red, averaging about 0.5 liters per person per week (or about one glass per day). The Cannonau grapes native to that region produce more red pigment, which contributes to the battle against harsh UV rays. During wine production, the grapes are allowed to macerate longer than for other wines. The pigment and the maceration time result in two to three times greater levels of flavonoids than other wines.

The Sardinian diet, which includes a fair amount of cheese and some meat, looks nothing like the traditional Okinawan one, which is centered around sweet potatoes. Still, they make the cheese with milk from grass-fed sheep, and they often reserved the meat only for special occasions; hence, the overall diet is fairly low in meat. In general, meals are accompanied by plenty of whole-grain bread, beans, vegetables, and (almost always) a glass of red wine. These are, of course, the hallmarks of the oft-exalted Mediterranean diet.

Longevity Checklist: Sardinia

- ✓ **Calorie restriction/fasting:** Sardinians have "frugal" diets.
- ✓ **mTOR:** The diets are low in animal protein with emphasis on vegetables and legumes.
- ✓ **Tea/coffee/wine:** Like most Italians, they drink plenty of red wine.
- ✓ **Salt:** They have high sodium intake from milk and cheese.
- ✓ **Fat:** They eat lots of chestnuts and walnuts, which are high in monounsaturated fats. The diet is higher in dairy fats.

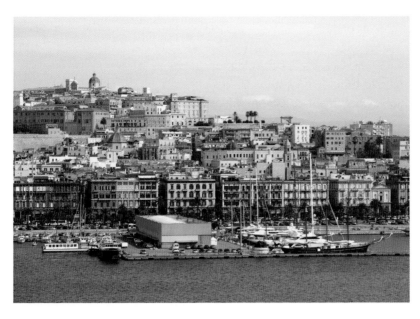

Loma Linda, California

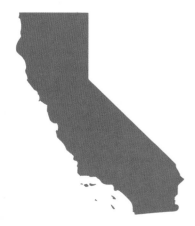

Loma Linda, California, which is just 60 miles east of the sprawling metropolis of Los Angeles, is an unlikely place to find one of the world's highest rates of longevity. Its residents, who live as much as a decade longer than the average American, largely belong to the Seventh-day Adventist Church, a theology that recommends vegetarianism and abstinence from smoking and alcohol.

Loma Linda University, operated by the Seventh-day Adventist Church, first began its study of the dietary and lifestyle habits of close to 25,000 residents in 1960. The original study, the Adventist Mortality Study (1960 to 1965), showed a significantly lower rate of cancer and heart disease compared to non-Adventists in the United States, which translated into a longevity advantage of 6.2 years for men and 3.7 years for women. The next study, the Adventist Health Study I (1974 to 1988), confirmed this finding; Adventist men lived 7.3 years more than the average Californian and women lived 4.4 years longer. The five main behaviors to which researchers attributed the benefits were not smoking, regular exercise, maintaining healthy body weight, eating more nuts, and eating a plant-based diet.

Although there is no controversy about the first three behaviors being healthy, the importance of eating nuts, which are high in natural fats, was highly controversial at the time the results were published. Since then, multiple other studies have confirmed those results. Although much of the benefits in the Adventist study in the popular press has been ascribed to the plant-based diet, it is likely the lack of tobacco use that is the most important factor.

The latest major Adventist Health Study (AHS-2), which started in 2002 and is ongoing, has analyzed the diets of 96,000 church members around North America. So far, the researchers have concluded that those members who've followed a vegetarian diet (a little more than half the population) are less likely to develop high cholesterol, high blood pressure, diabetes, metabolic syndrome, and even various types of cancer.[10] In particular, Adventists who eat more fruits, legumes, and tomatoes have shown lower rates of certain cancers.[11]

Longevity Checklist: Loma Linda

- ☑ **Calorie restriction/fasting:** Residents of Loma Linda eat a vegetarian diet that's often lower in calories than a diet that includes meat.
- ☑ **mTOR:** Residents of Loma Linda eat a diet high in plant protein and low in animal protein.
- ◯ **Tea/coffee/wine:** Tea and coffeeare not specifically encouraged or prohibited. (The Adventists do not drink alcohol.)
- ◯ **Salt:** The diet includes a normal level of salt.
- ☑ **Fat:** The diet includes nuts, which means people consume a high level of natural fats.

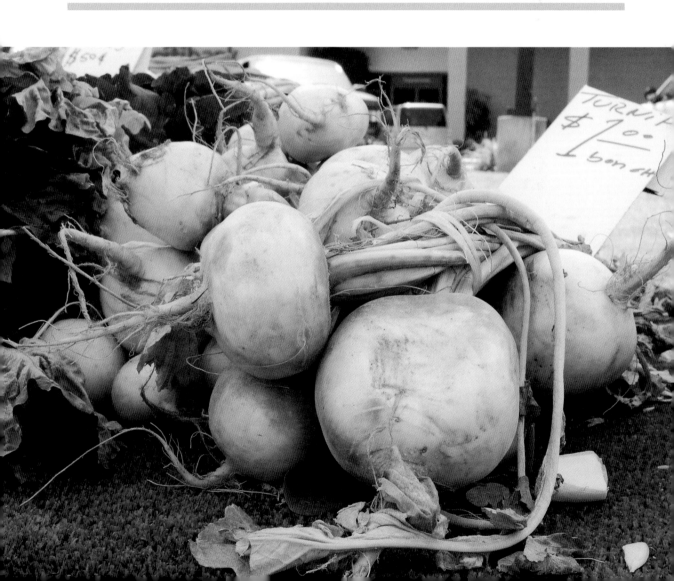

Nicoya Peninsula, Costa Rica

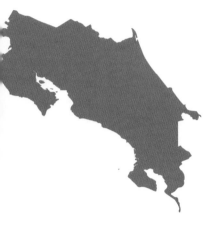

Further south, along the sunny northern Pacific coast of Costa Rica, lies the Nicoya region. Its residents, especially the men, reach the age of 90 at a rate 2.5 times greater than people in the United States.[12] The probability of a 60-year-old Nicoyan man celebrating his 100th birthday is seven times that of a Japanese and Sardinian male, and he has a lower risk of cardiovascular disease.

The traditional Nicoyan diet is high in fiber; it's largely plant-based with staple foods like freshly made corn tortillas, black beans, papayas, bananas, and yams. Nicoyans might eat chicken, pork, and beef, but mostly their plates are filled with starches like rice and beans.[13] They do consume slightly more calories, carbohydrates, proteins, and fiber than the average Costa Rican, who also rank fairly high on the longevity spectrum. Nicoyans' protein intake is 73 grams per day, which is much lower than the 100 grams of the average American. Overall, the residents of the Nicoya peninsula tend to stick to their traditional foods rather than eating processed and refined varieties.

Longevity Checklist: Nicoya Peninsula

- ✓ **Calorie restriction/fasting:** Nicoyans eat a plant-based diet that's typically very low in overall calories. They tend to eat very little in the evening.
- ✓ **mTOR:** Nicoyans eat a plant-based diet that is low in meat.
- ✓ **Tea/coffee/wine:** Nicoyans are heavy coffee drinkers. They usually drink it daily.
- ○ **Salt:** Nicoyans eat a normal amount of salt.
- ✓ **Fat:** Because of the vegetable-based diet, Nicoyans have a lower fat intake overall, but they get some fat from animal sources. They do not use vegetable oils.

Ikaria, Greece

The small, mountainous island of Ikaria, named for the legend of Icarus, sits in the Aegean Sea between the mainland of Greece and Turkey. Its population of nearly 8,500 inhabitants follows mostly Greek Orthodox Christian traditions. They live to be 90 years old around three times as often as Americans, and many are unaffected by dementia and age-related chronic diseases.[14] Ikaria's reputation as a health destination dates back 2,500 years; the ancient Greeks would travel to this small island to soak in the hot springs.

Anyone following a Mediterranean-style diet should look straight to the plate of the Ikarians, who eat an abundance of fresh fruits and vegetables, whole grains, beans, potatoes, and plenty of olive oil. They also indulge in antioxidant-rich herbal teas of wild rosemary, sage, and oregano. A typical breakfast consisted of bread and honey with wine, coffee, or a local mountain tea. Lunch was almost always beans (lentils, garbanzo) and local, seasonal vegetables. Dinner was typically bread and goat's milk. Ikarians would eat meat on special occasions.[15] The local Ikarian diet, typical of other Mediterranean diets, included plenty of olive oil, wine, and vegetables, and it's lower in meat protein than other Western diets. On average, Ikarians eat fish twice per week, and they eat meat only five times per month. They frequently drink coffee (averaging 2 to 3 cups per day) and wine (about 2 to 3.5 glasses per day). Ikarians consume only about a quarter of the refined sugar that Americans eat. Bread tends to be sourdough, although they also eat stone ground wheat bread. Probably more importantly, one resident notes that "Food is always enjoyed in combination with conversation."[16]

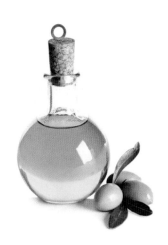

As devout Greek Orthodox Christians, many Ikarians also follow a religious calendar that includes many periods of fasting. One study that looked at fasting in particular found that those who regularly fasted reported lower blood cholesterol and body mass index (BMI).[17] Of course, we already know the other impressive benefits that come with calorie restriction and fasting, including reduced blood pressure, cholesterol, the risk of several chronic diseases, and the potential to live a much longer, healthier life.

Longevity Checklist: Ikaria

✓ **Calorie restriction/fasting:** Ikarians follow the Greek Orthodox tradition of fasting.

✓ **mTOR:** Ikarians eat a diet low in animal protein.

✓ **Tea/coffee/wine:** Ikarians drink lots of coffee and red wine.

✓ **Salt:** There are natural salt springs in Therma. The diet includes high levels of salt from milk, cheese, and olives.

✓ **Fat:** The sources of fat include lots of olive oil and fish.

The UnBlue Zone: The Southern United States

In contrast to the healthy Blue Zones, certain diets in parts of the world are associated with increased risk of heart disease and decreased longevity. It is just as useful to look at these diets to learn what *not* to do as it is to look at the Blue Zones to determine what to do. The best-studied example comes from the southeastern area of the United States. The Reasons for Geographic and Racial Differences in Stroke (REGARDS) study[18] followed more than 17,000 adult participants over five years to look at various dietary patterns, including a so-called "Southern diet." The Southern pattern of eating was high in fried foods and added fats (mostly vegetable oils), eggs, organ meats, processed meats, and sugar-sweetened beverages. Where most diet patterns studied were neutral on cardiovascular health, the Southern diet stood out as especially harmful to human health, with a huge 56 percent increase in the risk of cardiovascular disease, 50 percent increase in kidney disease, and 30 percent increase in stroke. This group also had more obesity, high blood pressure, and type 2 diabetes than the rest of the United States.

The Southern diet was not particularly high in calories; the average was about 1,500 calories per day. The macronutrient composition also wasn't particularly different from the rest of the United States—about 50 percent carbohydrates and 35 percent fat. This finding emphasizes that we must do more than look at the general categories of macronutrients; we also must look at specific foods for their effect.

The total amount of red meat in the Southern diet was not particularly high, but the quantities of processed meats were off the charts. There is a huge difference between rib eye steak and a hot dog. The processing of meat introduces numerous chemicals and other additives (such as sugar, sweeteners, nitrates, and phosphates) that may adversely affect health. Also, the Southern dietary pattern contained large amounts of bread.

The Southern Diet is an example of a diet that does not promote longevity. There is no calorie restriction or fasting, and the high sugar intake means that insulin levels are high, which contributes to the excessive obesity rates that are common in the southeast United States. Indeed, the three most obese states in the United States in 2014 were Mississippi, West Virginia, and Louisiana.

The relatively high American meat consumption means that mTOR is kept high. Instead of eating natural fats, the Southern diet includes added fats, almost all of which are vegetable oils. People commonly cook fried foods in industrial seed oils, which are inexpensive and readily available.

Longevity Checklist: Southern U.S.

- ○ **Calorie restriction/fasting:** The Southern diet doesn't include any calorie restriction or fasting. The usual American dietary advice is to eat more than three times per day.
- ○ **mTOR:** The Southern diet is high in meats and processed meats.
- ○ **Tea/coffee/wine:** There's no specific emphasis on these beverages in this diet. People drink iced tea, but it's very high in sugar.
- ⊘ **Salt:** This diet is high in salt, mostly from processed foods.
- ○ **Fat:** Vegetable oils are a prominent part of this diet.

What If You Don't Live in a Blue Zone?

The Blue Zone areas share more than just diet. In this book, we've focused intentionally on dietary determinants of longevity, but there is more to it than that. A healthy dose of sun and sea, some mountainous terrain, and a dedication to natural movement are integral to the longevity of people in these areas. The healthiest people in the world don't go to the gym. They don't sweat to the oldies. They don't use a treadmill. They don't pump iron. They don't run marathons. They include movement as part of their natural way of life.

In these Blue Zones, movement is life. People walk. They climb mountains, not because they are there but to tend their sheep. They tend their gardens. They dance. They play games: soccer when they're young and lawn bowling when they're older. They don't use stand-up desks. The healthiest people not only eat natural foods but they follow natural movements. When sharks stop swimming, they die. When people stop moving, we, too, die a little at a time.

Socializing and maintaining tight-knit communities also plays a significant role in longevity. The healthiest people in the world don't eat in front of the TV. They eat with their family and friends. They linger over shared meals because they are enjoyable. They don't grab a quick bite simply to eat.

What lessons can you learn from people in Blue Zones if you're not lucky enough to live in one? Keeping insulin, calories, and mTOR low is a great start. You can do this with plant-based diets, but none of the Blue Zones are completely vegetarian or vegan; each includes some animal foods. This fact is important to note because there is a risk for vitamin A and vitamin B12 deficiency on a vegan diet if you don't use appropriate supplementation. Vegetarians and vegans eat more fiber and less protein on average—and little to no animal protein. A French study finds that vegetarians and vegans ate 33 percent and 75 percent more fiber than meat-eaters, respectively, but both groups eat fewer overall calories, total protein, and fats.[19]

Although many Blue Zones share this plant-based diet, this is not proof that eating plants is healthier than eating meat. It's possible that meat was limited in the diets of these areas not by choice but simply because people couldn't afford to eat a meat-based diet. Many other areas of the world also eat a primarily plant-based diet without having a specific longevity advantage. For example, many people in India eat a vegetarian diet, yet the life expectancy of Indian citizens in 2018 ranked 165th in the world at an unremarkable 69.1 years. Eating meat is not necessarily unhealthy; Hong Kong has now surpassed the rest of Asia in longevity although its residents eat a diet comparatively high in meat. As in life, the importance is balance. Eating sufficient meat is just as important as avoiding excessive meat intake.

Eating a plant-based diet does not guarantee that the diet is healthy, just as eating a meat-based diet does not guarantee that it's unhealthy. The key is eating the *right* vegetables and meats. Vegetarians in the Adventist Health Study typically increased their consumption of fruits, vegetables, avocados, whole grains, legumes, soy, nuts, and seeds while reducing their intake of refined grains, added fats, sweets, snack foods, and non-water beverages. Eating a chocolate donut can be 100 percent vegan. Drinking sugary soda is 100 percent vegan. Eating potato chips (fried in vegetable oil) is 100 percent vegan. But few would argue that eating and drinking these things are inherently healthy just because they are of plant origin. Long-term maintenance of a vegetarian or low-meat diet can reduce the risk of diabetes, cancer, hypertension, cardiovascular diseases, and mortality from all causes if you do it properly.[20] If you do it improperly—using refined grains, refined vegetable oils, and sugars—a vegetarian diet may be a health nightmare.

As far as total protein intake, if you follow the traditional Mediterranean diet of the Sardinians and Ikarians—which does allow for some animal products—you'd still be consuming only about 15 percent total protein and 43 percent carbohydrates.[21] Or if you want to take lessons from the Okinawan centenarians, you'd be reserving only about 9 percent of your diet for protein with a whopping 85 percent for carbohydrates.

Less Protein, Longer Life?

We can't eliminate protein, of course. Too little protein at any age can lead to malnutrition. As we age, protein becomes just as crucial as it was when we were younger—just for different reasons. Most elderly people don't get enough protein to maintain a strong, healthy muscle mass. A lack of certain amino acids, like cysteine (a crucial player in the body's internal antioxidant system), can also promote aging and oxidative stress.

Calorie restriction and fasting have long been proven as likely tools for longevity, but the intricacies behind why is still a mystery. Balance, of course, is essential, and being mindful of the type and amount of protein—and carbohydrates—you consume could be the key to a longer, healthier life. Promises of longevity are complicated; IGF-1 and mTOR, both of which promote growth, could be significant factors (refer to Chapter 3). Reducing protein consumption has been shown to lower both IGF-1 and mTOR, even lowering IGF-1 significantly in just three weeks.

Unfortunately, we can't give you any exact numbers that tell you the magical amount of macronutrients to guarantee a long, disease-free life. From the evidence we have now, we can propose that a normal, healthy person should consume anywhere from 1.0 to 1.8 grams of protein per kilogram of body weight per day. Where you fall in that range depends on myriad factors—your current age, health, activity level, and even your overall diet itself.

Importantly, quantity is *not* the only variable that matters. Quality and the source of protein—animal versus plant—may be just as significant as the proteins themselves. We can look to the healthy centenarians in the Blue Zones of Okinawa, Sardinia, Loma Linda, Nikoya, or Ikaria for some real-life evidence and inspiration. Their traditional, largely plant-based and lower-protein diets have kept their populations living longer and healthier for centuries. But even in some of these areas, those eating patterns are quickly fading, and so are their enviable health and longevity stats, thanks to some unfortunate Western-inspired habits.

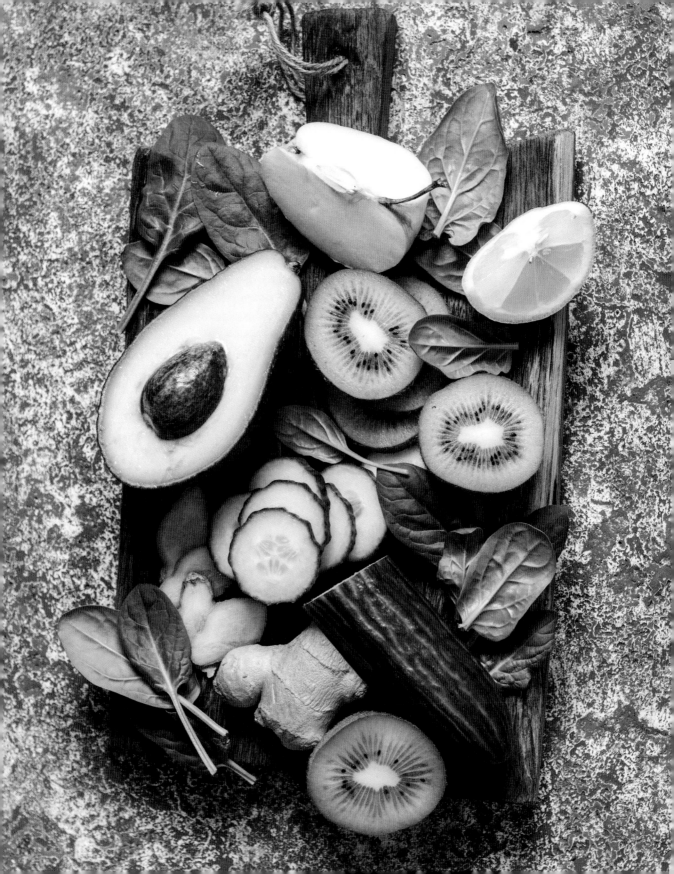

13

FULL PLAN FOR HEALTHY AGING

There is no single secret to healthy aging and longevity. As discussed in Chapter 12, those people who live in the various Blue Zones have taken completely different paths to living past 100 years of age. But all these people share some common dietary practices. In this chapter, we outline five steps that make up our *Longevity Solution* checklist. Following most, if not all, of these steps, may dramatically improve your overall health.

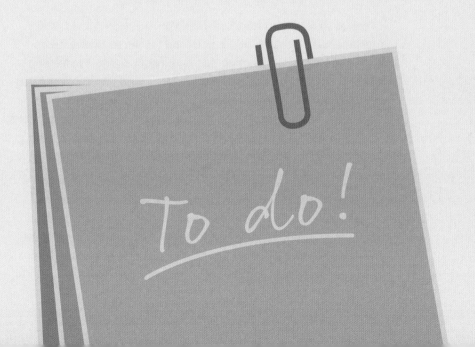

Step 1: CalorieRestriction/ Fasting

Calorie restriction has the potential to increase longevity and improve health, but it's very difficult to implement in daily practice. Certainly, there has been no shortage of ways we've tried to reduce calories, including mandatory calorie labels and calorie counting books and apps. The Okinawans demonstrate that it's possible to follow a plan of deliberate calorie restriction, but they remind themselves daily to do this by stopping before being full. A more practical solution may be fasting. Intermittent fasting has almost as many variations as there are practitioners. With intermittent fasting, you can decrease protein intake without altering much of anything about the food you eat.

Prolonged fasting—which is fasting for more than twenty-four hours but not more than once per two weeks unless you're part of a special patient population and being closely monitored by a physician—might have profound antiaging effects. However, you should not perform prolonged fasting too frequently to preserve lean body mass and mineral status.

The following are some of the fasting intervals:

- **Twelve to fourteen hours of fasting:** You restrict food intake for twelve to fourteen hours and feed for ten to twelve hours per day (usually consuming just two meals during the feeding period). When you eat, your body stores food energy. When you fast, your body burns food energy. Therefore, maintaining an even balance is essential for everyday life. This was the standard eating pattern for Americans up to the 1970s. You follow this schedule by reducing or eliminating late-night feedings.

- **16:8 intermittent fast:** You restrict food intake for sixteen hours and feed for eight hours per day (usually consuming just two meals during the feeding period). Many people find skipping breakfast and eating a larger lunch and dinner to be the easiest way to follow an intermittent fast schedule. This schedule is also called *time-restricted eating*.

- **Alternate day fasting:** On one day, you eat one meal, optimally between noon and 2:00 p.m. This is a 24-hour fasting period, which is a schedule that's sometimes called *one meal a day*. The following day, you follow a normal schedule of feeding. You generally do this two to three times per week.

- **Prolonged fast:** You fast more than twenty-four hours at a time. It's best to undertake prolonged fasting with medical supervision.

For more details on the practical aspects of fasting, see *The Complete Guide to Fasting: Heal Your Body Through Intermittent, Alternate-Day, and Extended Fasting*, coauthored by Dr. Fung.

Step 2: mTOR/Protein

There are several determinants of optimal protein intake. You must decide what amount of protein is appropriate for you and what you need for growth. (See Chapter 9 for specific details.) When you know what amount of protein to consume, you then need to determine what sources you'll use. Protein is not a stand-alone nutrient; it is found in food, and, except for protein supplements, other nutrients (carbohydrate and/or fat) always accompany it. Anyone who decides to alter his or her protein intake, whether higher or lower, needs to know which foods are high or low in protein.

Animal foods—meat, fish, dairy, and eggs—have the highest protein content. Manipulating protein intake higher or lower usually means changing the amount of animal foods you eat. Eggs and fish contain the highest amount of protein as a percentage of calories; butter and cream are the only two animal foods that contain little to no protein.

Red meat, pork, chicken, and fish contain about 6 to 9 grams of protein per ounce, so a small 3-ounce serving contains about 18 to 27 grams of protein. If you're an average adult man, this is already about one-third of the protein you need in an entire day. A large egg contains about 8 grams of protein, so three eggs at a meal get you to around one-third your required intake.

The Atkins diet is the prototypical low-carbohydrate weight-loss diet. Although it doesn't require high protein, that is normally the outcome for people who follow this diet. The Atkins diet recommends eating large amounts of meat, cheese, eggs, and other animal foods. For those who want to restrict protein but still eat a low-carbohydrate diet or to lose weight, there are other ways of eating that are just as effective. The so-called Eco-Atkins diet has been shown in clinical trials to be effective for weight loss and in lowering LDL cholesterol. The Eco-Atkins diet is entirely vegan (no animal foods), and protein comes from gluten, soy, vegetables, and nuts. The Low Carb High Fat (LCHF) diet specifically reduces carbohydrates but keeps protein moderate. Ketogenic diets are also examples of LCHF diets because high protein can prevent ketosis.

Vegan diets are those that eliminate all animal foods. For someone desiring to lower protein consumption, that's a good thing, but there could be a danger of not getting enough protein, something also to be avoided during periods of growth. Those who follow the vegan lifestyle but want more protein need to consider their food choices carefully. Beans average about 15 grams of protein per cup, but vegetables have only about 1 or 2 grams per ounce.

Protein supplements might be useful for those who want to have more protein, such as athletes or the elderly and ill. Besides providing concentrated protein, whey has several health benefits. Other choices for protein supplementation include casein, soy, pea, and rice.

The following are recommended protein intakes for adults performing resistance versus nonresistance training:

- **Resistance training:** Aim for 1.6 to 2.2 grams of protein per kilogram of body weight per day.

- **Nonresistance training:** Aim for 1.2 grams of protein per kilogram of body weight per day.

Use the following guidelines to decide how to get protein and determine whether to use animal or plant sources:

- Aim to obtain 50 percent of your protein intake from animal sources and 50 percent from plant sources (although you can alter this to a range of up to 25 percent plant sources to 75 percent animal sources or vice versa).

- Try to use organic sources of protein. For animal protein sources, look for foods sourced as close to nature as possible, such as pasture-raised for butter, eggs, dairy, and meat. Feedlot cattle (fed grain) have a very different fat profile than grass-fed beef.

- Aim to get half of your animal protein from marine sources (oysters, fish, shellfish, and so on).

- Use a variety of plant protein sources, such as spinach, onions, garlic, cooked and cooled potatoes (to quadruple the resistant starch), and beans.

Specific supplements are useful in some cases. Traditional societies in which people ate "nose-to-tail" often obtained adequate amounts of the amino acid glycine from the collagen in tendons, joints, and skin. If your diet does not include these sources, then you might consider adding hydrolyzed collagen at a dose of 20 to 60 grams per day and/or a glycine supplement in the form of powders or capsules at a dose of glycine of 10 to 15 grams per day.

Step 3: Coffee, Tea, and Wine

Most of us in North America don't need to be told twice to enjoy a good cup of Joe. The successes of coffee chains like Starbucks are evidence of coffee's hold on us. Luckily, we can enjoy our coffee guilt-free because we know that there are many healthful compounds in coffee. Drinking between one and five cups per day seems best, and you can vary the amount according to your preferences.

We need to offer a few cautions, however. Avoid drinking coffee with sugar or other sweeteners. Adding 1 or 2 teaspoons of sugar to your coffee will quickly add up if you drink five cups per day. A small amount of cream or milk is adequate. Choose an organic coffee. Caffeinated coffee may have certain advantages over decaffeinated coffee for a reduction in waist circumference and visceral fat loss, but it has the unfortunate downside of inducing several side effects, such as increased urination and jitteriness. It might be best to drink coffee with meals to reduce the absorption of iron. Also, the polyphenols in coffee can help reduce the oxidative stress that may come with a meal.

Tea is also a great beverage choice. Green tea, with its high dose of catechins, might be the longevity secret of much of the Asian subcontinent. Black and oolong teas contain many other flavonoids that may be similarly beneficial. Drink teas plentifully throughout the day. Try Pique Tea crystals (www.piquetea.com); that brand uses a cold brew crystallization process that yields up to three times the amount of catechins in green tea.

Research of numerous cultures has uncovered that red wine is consistently associated with longevity. The main benefits of drinking daily moderate amounts of red wine likely do not come from the alcohol content but the polyphenols in red wine, such as quercetin and resveratrol. Consuming high resveratrol wines may provide enhanced cardiovascular benefits. Importantly, you should consume red wine only in moderate amounts (two drinks for men, one drink for women) and take it with your largest meal of the day. For certain people, alcohol can be addictive; it can be a slippery slope for individuals to consume only one or two drinks (anywhere from 3 to 10 ounces) of red wine per day.

The following are some recommendations of what you should look for when choosing a wine:

- Preferably a high-resveratrol wine such as Brazilian, Pinot Noir, or Lambrusco

- Preferably low in sugar such as Dry Farm Wines

- Preferably an organic version to avoid pesticide contamination in your wine

Furthermore, use these guidelines for consuming wine:

- Consume wine with the largest meal of the day

- Consume wine daily (6 ounces for men and 3 ounces for women) rather than binge drinking

Step 4: Salt—Sodium and Magnesium

Your body naturally requires about 4 grams of sodium (2 teaspoons) of salt per day. Deliberately restricting this essential mineral leads to numerous health consequences, including insulin resistance, kidney and adrenal dysfunction, muscle spasms, dehydration, and magnesium and calcium deficiency. Eat your salt with real food and make sure you choose a high-quality salt such as Redmond Real Salt (www.realsalt.com), which comes from an ancient underground ocean. Salts from underground ancient dried up oceans lack the microplastics and heavy metals that can contaminate nearly all sea salts from modern-day oceans. Additionally, Redmond Real Salt has good amounts of iodine and calcium in it, which can help to replace those two minerals that you lose in sweat during exercise or trips to the sauna.

When it comes to magnesium, you should be picky about the supplement you choose. Many commercial magnesium supplements are magnesium oxide, which is the cheapest form to produce. However, magnesium oxide is poorly absorbed in the gastrointestinal system compared to magnesium diglycinate (also called glycinate) and magnesium citrate. Magnesium chloride also appears to have good absorption; however, the intake of chloride without sodium can pose some additional problems, especially if it's not balanced with bicarbonate (because chloride is acidic). Most of the population is not getting enough magnesium to hit optimal intakes. In fact, almost everyone should be supplementing with around 300 milligrams of magnesium each day in some form or another (such as high-magnesium mineral waters or supplements).

The following are recommendations for salt and magnesium intake:

- Choose a high-quality salt such as Redmond Real Salt.
- Take salt before and during exercise, especially when exercising in the heat. See Dr. DiNicolantonio's book *The Salt Fix* for a detailed description of how much salt to take before and during exercise.
- Supplement with around 300 milligrams of magnesium from either high-magnesium mineral waters or high-quality magnesium diglycinate or magnesium citrate supplements.

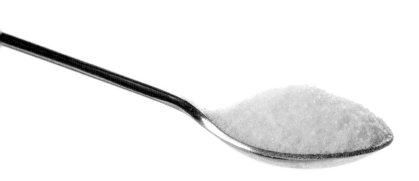

Step 5: Eat More Natural, Healthy Fats

Your healthy fats should come in the form of wild seafood such as sardines, salmon, shrimp, oysters, lobster, mussels, clams, and crab. These sources of protein should make up about half of your animal protein intake to ensure an optimal intake of long-chain omega-3s as well as giving you the additional benefit of providing the antioxidant astaxanthin. If you cannot afford wild seafood, or you simply don't like the taste of it, consider supplemental krill oil, algal oil, or fish oil (or some combination of them). Krill oil has the benefit of having astaxanthin in it, which can help protect the highly susceptible polyunsaturated fats in your brain from oxidizing. You might want to limit your intake of wild seafood to twice per week because of persistent organic pollutants and heavy metals. The other five days of the week you can supplement with krill oil and fish oil to boost your omega-3 status without the risk of contamination.

Avoid industrial trans fats and industrial seed oils. In the real world, this means avoiding most packaged foods that have a long list of ingredients, especially donuts and other deep-fried doughs. Almost all packaged foods contain large amounts of hidden omega-6 seed oils, so be sure to read food labels and avoid anything that contains soybean, sunflower, corn, cottonseed, or safflower oil.

The other half of your animal protein intake should come from pastured eggs, grass-fed dairy and cheese, and pastured or grass-fed meats. Regular meat and dairy are reasonable if the grass-fed alternatives are unavailable. However, be careful of factory-farmed eggs; they are nothing like pastured eggs, and you should keep them to a minimum in your diet. To reduce the oxidation of the omega-6 and cholesterol in eggs, you should cook them over easy or over medium; do not scramble them. Using pastured butter for cooking, as long as you cook at a low heat to prevent or reduce the oxidation of cholesterol, is a healthy way to cook. Pasteurized and ultra-pasteurized cow's milk likely contains oxidized cholesterol; hence, you should limit your intake of cow's milk to moderate amounts. A healthier alternative may be organic coconut milk.

Here are some guidelines to use for making sure you get the right kinds of healthy fats in your life:

- Consume around 2 to 4 grams of EPA and DHA per day from wild seafood, but limit wild fish to twice a week unless it comes from a clean source such as Alaska or Canada.
- Consider taking a high-quality krill oil supplement (up to 4 grams per day) plus a high-quality algal oil or fish oil supplement (up to 4 grams of EPA/DHA per day).
- Consume plant omega-3s from chia, hemp, or flax seeds. Target an intake of 30 to 60 grams (1 to 2 ounces) per day.
- Feel free to eat and cook with animal fats (pastured butter, ghee, tallow, lard, etc.).
- Omega-6 fats should come from whole foods (nuts, seeds, pastured eggs, and chicken). Keep the omega-6 to omega-3 ratio at 4 or less.
- Consume 1 to 2 tablespoons of organic extra-virgin olive oil, or a handful of organic olives, per day.
- See Dr. DiNicolantonio's book *Superfuel: Ketogenic Keys to Unlock the Secrets of Good Fats, Bad Fats, and Great Health* for a deeper dive into good fats versus bad fats. You also can visit his website at http://drjamesdinic.com.

For more details about healthy fats, see Dr. DiNicolantonio's book *Superfuel: Ketogenic Keys to Unlock the Secrets of Good Fats, Bad Fats, and Great Health.*

THE *LONGEVITY SOLUTION* DIETARY PYRAMID

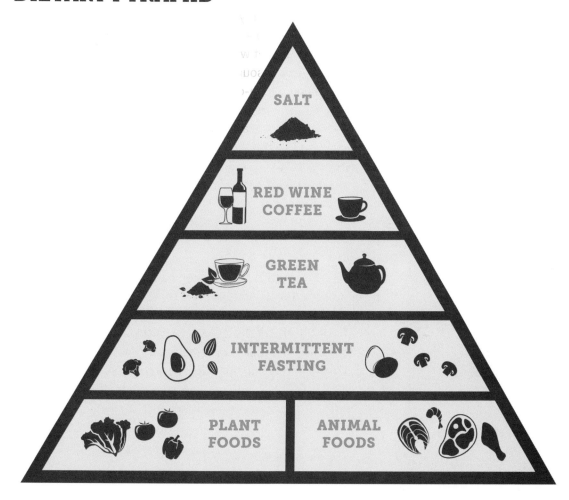

SALT

RED WINE
COFFEE

GREEN
TEA

INTERMITTENT
FASTING

PLANT
FOODS

ANIMAL
FOODS

EPILOGUE

Aging is a potent promoter of disease; rates of ill health rise precipitously with every decade past the age of maturity. Dietary protein, which provides the necessary material for growth, is intimately connected to aging, a consequence of the trade-off between growth and longevity.

Animal foods, which contain large amounts of protein, typically cost more than plant foods. Here, we're talking about cost in money as well as in the energy and effort our ancestors spent tracking and hunting down an animal versus simply pulling a potato from the ground or picking a few berries from a bush. Historically, people consumed meat much less than grains and other plant foods. However, modern methods of food production have made it possible for almost everybody to consume more than enough meat and other animal foods. Excessive protein intake, especially from animal products, may drive aging. Excessive protein intake is now more of a concern than it was in the past when underconsumption of protein was the main problem.

For years, experts have advised us to lower our consumption of saturated fat, which is mainly found in animal foods, and that advice seems increasingly misguided. However, until recently, little consideration had been given to the amount of protein we consume. New research has shown how the biochemical mechanisms of growth, exemplified by mTOR and IGF-1, also promote aging. Calorie restriction, the most potent lifespan-extension intervention known, also restricts protein, a factor that accounts for a great deal of fasting's antiaging effect. Although few people are willing or able to restrict their calories over long periods of time, close attention to the amount of protein consumed could provide much of the benefit of restricting calories.

At the same time, targeted use of extra and different types of protein can help the ill and elderly maintain muscle and prevent frailty, keeping them out of a state of dependence that often requires full-time care in a nursing home. More protein also is required by those who exercise regularly. Perhaps most importantly, increasing the intake of glycine might reduce a person's need to restrict dietary protein to a large degree.

Living longer requires that the body invest resources in maintenance and repair. As we grow older, we can coax our bodies into more investment in the processes that help us live longer; keeping protein intake within bounds does this. Low IGF-1 production and mTOR might decrease the risk of cancer and other diseases, but protein restriction also can go too far. Cysteine and glycine help increase the antioxidant glutathione in the body. Not eating too much protein but also getting enough for vital functions of the body is a slippery slope.

Until now, we've given little consideration to the primary physiological drivers of aging, which are connected to protein intake. Optimizing both protein quantity and the source of protein increases the odds of healthy aging. Add in other well-known healthy practices—such as exercise; intermittent fasting; avoiding processed junk foods; eating natural, unprocessed foods; and consuming green tea, coffee, red wine, high-quality salts, omega-3s, glycine, collagen, and magnesium—and you have a powerful recipe for longevity.

ENDNOTES

Chapter 1

1. Olshansky, S. J., et al. "A Potential Decline in Life Expectancy in the United States in the 21st Century." *New England Journal of Medicine* 352, no. 11 (2005): 1138–45.
2. "Life Expectancy in the USA, 1900–98." Accessed at *http://u.demog.berkeley.edu/~andrew/1918/figure2.html.*
3. Tippett, R. "Mortality and Cause of Death, 1900 v. 2010." Carolina Demography, June 16, 2014. Accessed at *http://demography.cpc.unc.edu/2014/06/16/mortality-and-cause-of-death-1900-v-2010/.*
4. "Statistical Fact Sheet, 2013 Update: Older Americans & Cardiovascular Diseases."American Heart Association. Accessed at *www.heart.org/idc/groups/heart-public/@wcm/@sop/@smd/documents/downloadable/ucm_319574.pdf.*
5. "Cancer Incidence Statistics." Cancer Research UK. Accessed at *www.cancerresearchuk.org/health-professional/cancer-statistics/incidence/age - heading-Zero.*
6. De Grey, A. "Life Span Extension Research and Public Debate: Societal Considerations." *Studies in Ethics, Law, and Technology* 1, no. 1 (2007).
7. "Using Yeast in Biology." Your Genome. Accessed at *www.yourgenome.org/stories/using-yeast-in-biology.*
8. Kachroo, A. H., et al. "Evolution. Systematic Humanization of Yeast Genes Reveals Conserved Functions and Genetic Modularity." *Science* 348, no. 6237 (2015): 921–5.
9. "Why Mouse Matters." National Human Genome Research Institute, July 23, 2010. Accessed at *www.genome.gov/10001345/.*
10. Kirkwood, T. B., and R. Holliday. "The Evolution of Ageing and Longevity." *Proceedings of the Royal Society B: Biological Sciences* 205, no. 1161 (1979): 531–46.
11. Kirkwood, T. B. "Understanding the Odd Science of Aging." *Cell* 120, no. 4 (2005): 437–47.
12. Ristow, M., et al. "Antioxidants Prevent Health-Promoting Effects of Physical Exercise in Humans." *Proceedings of the National Academy of Sciences of the United States of America* 106, no. 21 (2009): 8665–70.
13. Pak, J. W., et al. "Rebuttal to Jacobs: The Mitochondrial Theory of Aging: Alive and Well." *Aging Cell* 2, no. 1 (2003): 9–10.
14. Rasmussen, U. F., et al. "Experimental Evidence Against the Mitochondrial Theory of Aging. A Study of Isolated Human Skeletal Muscle Mitochondria." *Experimental Gerontology* 38, no. 8 (2003): 877–86.
15. Vermulst, M., et al. "Mitochondrial Point Mutations Do Not Limit the Natural Lifespan of Mice." *Nature Genetics* 39, no. 4 (2007): 540–3.
16. Inglis-Arkell, E. "The Ironic End of the Man Who Made Himself Immune to Poison." Gizmodo io9, January 4, 2013. Accessed at *https://io9.gizmodo.com/5972414/the-ironic-end-of-the-man-who-made-himself-immune-to-poison*; "King Mithradates VI of Pontus Used Poison to Avoid Death by Poison." Ancient Pages, March 5, 2016. Accessed at *www.ancientpages.com/2016/03/05/king-mithradates-vi-of-pontus-used-poison-to-avoid-death-by-poison/.*
17. Ibid.
18. Feinendegen, L. E. "Evidence for Beneficial Low Level Radiation Effects and Radiation Hormesis." *The British Journal of Radiology* 78, no. 925 (2005): 3–7.
19. Ibid.
20. Miller, R. A., et al. "Big Mice Die Young: Early Life Body Weight Predicts Longevity in Genetically Heterogeneous Mice." *Aging Cell* no. 1 (2002): 22–9.
21. He, Q., et al. "Shorter Men Live Longer: Association of Height with Longevity and FOXO3 Genotype in American Men of Japanese Ancestry." *PLoS One* 9, no. 5 (2014): e94385.
22. Blagosklonny, M. V. "Big Mice Die Young but Large Animals Live Longer." *Aging* (Albany, NY) 5, no. 4 (2013): 227–33.

Chapter 2

1. Masoro, E. J. "Overview of Caloric Restriction and Ageing." *Mechanisms of Ageing Development* 126, no. 9 (2005): 913–22.

2. McCay, C. M., et al. "The Effect of Retarded Growth upon the Length of Life Span and upon the Ultimate Body Size." *The Journal of Nutrition* 10, no. 1 (1935): 63–79.

3. Richardson, A., et al. "Significant Life Extension by Ten Percent Dietary Restriction." *Annals of the New York Academy of Science* 1363 (2016): 11–7.

4. Tannenbaum, A. "The Genesis and Growth of Tumors II. Effect of Caloric Restriction Per Se." *Cancer Research* 2, no. 7 (1942): 460–7.

5. Carlson, A. J., and F. Hoelzel. "Apparent Prolongation of the Life Span of Rats by Intermittent Fasting." *Journal of Nutrition* 31 (1946): 363–75.

6. Ross, M. H. "Protein, Calories and Life Expectancy." *Federation Proceedings* 18 (1959): 1190–207.

7. Iwasaki, K., et al. "The Influence of Dietary Protein Source on Longevity and Age-Related Disease Processes of Fischer Rats." *Journal of Gerontology* 43, no. 1 (1988): B5–12.

8. Redman, L. M., and E. Ravussin. "Caloric Restriction in Humans: Impact on Physiological, Psychological, and Behavioral Outcomes." *Antioxidants & Redox Signaling* 14, no. 2 (2011): 275–87; Suzuki, M., B. J. Wilcox, and C. D. Wilcox. "Implications from and for Food Cultures for Cardiovascular Disease: Longevity." *Asia Pacific Journal of Clinical Nutrition* 10, no. 2 (2001): 165–71.

9. Stanfel, M. N., et al. "The TOR Pathway Comes of Age." *Biochimica et Biophysica Acta* 1790, no. 10 (2009): 1067–74.

10. McDonald, R. B., and J. J. Ramsey. "Honoring Clive McCay and 75 Years of Calorie Restriction Research." *Journal of Nutrition* 140, no. 7 (2010): 1205–10.

11. Bluher, M. "Fat Tissue and Long Life." *Obesity Facts* 1, no. 4 (2008): 176–82.

12. Adelman, R., R. L. Saul, and B. N. Ames. "Oxidative Damage to DNA: Relation to Species Metabolic Rate and Life Span." *Proceedings of the National Academy of Sciences of the United States of America* 85, no. 8 (1988): 2706–8.

13. Hulbert, A. J., et al. "Life and Death: Metabolic Rate, Membrane Composition, and Life Span of Animals." *Physiological Reviews* 87, no. 4 (2007): 1175–213.

14. Mariotti, S., et al. "Complex Alteration of Thyroid Function in Healthy Centenarians." *Journal of Clinical Endocrinology and Metabolism* 77, no. 5 (1993): 1130–4.

15. See note 1 above.

16. Paolisso, G., et al. "Body Composition, Body Fat Distribution, and Resting Metabolic Rate in Healthy Centenarians." *American Journal of Clinical Nutrition* 62, no. 4 (1995): 746–50.

17. Lee, S. J., C. T. Murphy, and C. Kenyon. "Glucose Shortens the Life Span of C. elegans by Downregulating DAF-16/FOXO Activity and Aquaporin Gene Expression." *Cell Metabolism* 10, no. 5 (2009): 379–91.

18. Masoro, E. J., et al. "Dietary Restriction Alters Characteristics of Glucose Fuel Use." *Journal of Gerontology* 47, no. 6 (1992): B202–8.

19. Kenyon, C., et al. "A C. elegans Mutant That Lives Twice as Long as Wild Type." *Nature* 366, no. 6454 (1993): 461–4.

20. "Cynthia Kenyon." *https://en.wikipedia.org/wiki/Cynthia_Kenyon.*

21. Taubes, G. "Rare Form of Dwarfism Protects Against Cancer." *Discover*, March 27, 2013. Accessed at *http://discovermagazine.com/2013/april/19-double-edged-genes*.

22. Blagosklonny, M. V. "Calorie Restriction: Decelerating mTOR-Driven Aging from Cells to Organisms (Including Humans)." *Cell Cycle* 9, no. 4 (2010): 683–8.

23. Cuervo, A. M., et al. "Autophagy and Aging: The Importance of Maintaining 'Clean' Cells." *Autophagy* 1, no. 3 (2005): 131–40.

24. Jia, K., and B. Levine. "Autophagy Is Required for Dietary Restriction-Mediated Life Span Extension in C. elegans." *Autophagy* 3, no. 6 (2007): 597–9; Melendez, A., et al. "Autophagy Genes Are Essential for Dauer Development and Life-Span Extension in C. elegans." *Science* 301, no. 5638 (2003): 1387–91.

25. Alvers, A. L., et al. "Autophagy Is Required for Extension of Yeast Chronological Life Span by Rapamycin." *Autophagy* 5, no. 6 (2009): 847–9.

26. Hardie, D. G., F. A. Ross, and S. A. Hawley. "AMPK: A Nutrient and Energy Sensor That Maintains Energy Homeostasis." *Nature Reviews Molecular Cell Biology* 13, no. 4 (2012): 251–62.

27. Canto, C., and J. Auwerx. "Calorie Restriction: Is AMPK a Key Sensor and Effector?" *Physiology* (Bethesda) 26, no. 4 (2011): 214–24.

28. Lyons, C., and H. Roche. "Nutritional Modulation of AMPK-Impact upon Metabolic-Inflammation." *International Journal of Molecular Sciences* 19, no. 10 (2018): 3092.

29. Anson, R. M., B. Jones, and R. de Cabod. "The Diet Restriction Paradigm: A Brief Review of the Effects of Every-Other-Day Feeding." *Age* (Dordr) 27, no. 1 (2005): 17–25.

30. Hambly, C., et al. "Repletion of TNFalpha or Leptin in Calorically Restricted Mice Suppresses Post-Restriction Hyperphagia." *Disease Model Mechanisms* 5, no. 1 (2012): 83–94.

31. Goodrick, C. L., et al. "Effects of Intermittent Feeding upon Growth and Life Span in Rats." *Gerontology* 28, no. 4 (1982): 233–41.

32. Goldberg, E. L., et al. "Lifespan-Extending Caloric Restriction or mTOR Inhibition Impair Adaptive Immunity of Old Mice by Distinct Mechanisms." *Aging Cell* 14, no. 1 (2015): 130–8.

33. Ingram, D. K., et al. "Calorie Restriction Mimetics: An Emerging Research Field." *Aging Cell* 5, no. 2 (2006): 97–108.

Chapter 3

1. "Did a Canadian Medical Expedition Lead to the Discovery of an Anti-Aging Pill?" *Bloomberg News*, February 12, 2015. Accessed at *https://business.financialpost.com/news/did-a-canadian-medical-expedition-lead-to-the-discovery-of-an-anti-aging-pill.*

2. Mohsin, N., et al. "Complete Regression of Visceral Kaposi's Sarcoma After Conversion to Sirolimus." *Experimental and Clinical Transplantation* 3, no. 2 (2005): 366–9.

3. Blagosklonny, M. V. "Aging and Immortality: Quasi-Programmed Senescence and Its Pharmacologic Inhibition." *Cell Cycle* 5, no. 18 (2006): 2087–102.

4. Ortman, J., V. Velkoff, and H. Hogan. "An Aging Nation: The Older Population in the United States." May 2014. Accessed at *www.census.gov/prod/2014pubs/p25-1140.pdf.*

5. Christensen, K., et al. "Ageing Populations: The Challenges Ahead." *The Lancet* 374, no. 9696 (2009): 1196–208; Drachman, D. A. "Aging of the Brain, Entropy, and Alzheimer Disease." *Neurology* 67, no. 8 (2006): 1340–52; Holroyd, C., C. Cooper, and E. Dennison. "Epidemiology of Osteoporosis." *Best Practice & Research: Clinical Endocrinology & Metabolism* 22, no. 5 (2008): 671–85.

6. Nair, S., and J. Ren. "Autophagy and Cardiovascular Aging: Lesson Learned from Rapamycin." *Cell Cycle* 11, no. 11 (2012): 2092–9.

7. Powers, R. W., 3rd, et al. "Extension of Chronological Life Span in Yeast by Decreased TOR Pathway Signaling." *Genes & Development* 20, no. 2 (2006): 174–84.

8. Robida-Stubbs, S., et al. "TOR Signaling and Rapamycin Influence Longevity by Regulating SKN-1/Nrf and DAF-16/FoxO." *Cell Metabolism* 15, no. 5 (2012): 713–24.

9. Bjedov, I., et al. "Mechanisms of Life Span Extension by Rapamycin in the Fruit Fly Drosophila Melanogaster." *Cell Metabolism* 11, no. 1 (2010): 35–46.

10. Harrison, D., et al. "Rapamycin Fed Late in Life Extends Lifespan in Genetically Heterogeneous Mice." *Nature* 460 (2009): 392–5.

11. Halford, B. "Rapamycin's Secrets Unearthed." *Chemical & Engineering News* 94, no. 29 (2016): 26–30.

12. Urfer, S. R., et al. "A Randomized Controlled Trial to Establish Effects of Short-Term Rapamycin Treatment in 24 Middle-Aged Companion Dogs." *Geroscience* 39, no. 2 (2017): 117–27.

13. Lelegren, M., et al. "Pharmaceutical Inhibition of mTOR in the Common Marmoset: Effect of Rapamycin on Regulators of Proteostasis in a Non-Human Primate." *Pathobiology of Aging & Age Related Diseases* 6 (2016): 31793.

14. Spilman, P., et al. "Inhibition of mTOR by Rapamycin Abolishes Cognitive Deficits and Reduces Amyloid-Beta Levels in a Mouse Model of Alzheimer's Disease." *PLoS One* 5, no. 4 (2010): e9979.

15. Majumder, S., et al. "Lifelong Rapamycin Administration Ameliorates Age-Dependent Cognitive Deficits by Reducing IL-1beta and Enhancing NMDA Signaling." *Aging Cell* 11, no. 2 (2012): 326–35.

16. Liu, Y., et al. "Rapamycin-Induced Metabolic Defects Are Reversible in Both Lean and Obese Mice." *Aging* (Albany NY) 6, no. 9 (2014): 742–54.

17. Kolosova, N. G., et al. "Prevention of Age-Related Macular Degeneration-Like Retinopathy by Rapamycin in Rats." *American Journal of Pathology* 181, no. 2 (2012): 472–7.

18. Halloran, J., et al. "Chronic Inhibition of Mammalian Target of Rapamycin by Rapamycin Modulates Cognitive and Non-Cognitive Components of Behavior Throughout Lifespan in Mice." *Neuroscience* 223 (2012): 102–13; Tsai, P. T., et al. "Autistic-Like Behaviour and Cerebellar Dysfunction in Purkinje Cell Tsc1 Mutant Mice." *Nature* 488, no. 7413 (2012): 647–51; Perl, A. "mTOR Activation is a Biomarker and a Central Pathway to Autoimmune Disorders, Cancer, Obesity, and Aging." *Annals of the New York Academy of Science* 1346, no. 1 (2015): 33–44.

19. Mahe, E., et al. "Cutaneous Adverse Events in Renal Transplant Recipients Receiving Sirolimus-Based Therapy." *Transplantation* 79, no. 4 (2005): 476–82; McCormack, F. X., et al. "Efficacy and Safety of Sirolimus in

Lymphangioleiomyomatosis." *New England Journal of Medicine* 364, no. 17 (2011): 1595–606.

20. Mendelsohn, A. R., and J. W. Larrick. "Dissecting Mammalian Target of Rapamycin to Promote Longevity." *Rejuvenation Research* 15, no. 3 (2012): 334–7.

21. Johnston, O., et al. "Sirolimus Is Associated with New-Onset Diabetes in Kidney Transplant Recipients." *Journal of the American Society of Nephrology* 19, no. 7 (2008): 1411–8.

22. Lamming, D. W. "Inhibition of the Mechanistic Target of Rapamycin (mTOR)-Rapamycin and Beyond." *Cold Spring Harbor Perspectives in Medicine* 6, no. 5 (2016).

23. See note 20 above.

24. Arriola Apelo, S. I., et al. "Alternative Rapamycin Treatment Regimens Mitigate the Impact of Rapamycin on Glucose Homeostasis and the Immune System." *Aging Cell* 15, no. 1 (2016): 28–38.

25. See note 11 above.

26. Carlson, A. J., and F. Hoelzel. "Growth and Longevity of Rats Fed Omnivorous and Vegetarian Diets." *Journal of Nutrition* 34, no. 1 (1947): 81–96.

27. Siri-Tarino, P. W., et al. "Meta-Analysis of Prospective Cohort Studies Evaluating the Association of Saturated Fat with Cardiovascular Disease." *American Journal of Clinical Nutrition* 91, no. 3 (2010): 535–46.

28. "Background." National Cancer Institute Office of Cancer Clinical Proteomics Research. Accessed at *https://proteomics.cancer.gov/proteomics/ background.*

29. Speakman, J. R., S. E. Mitchell, and M. Mazidi. "Calories or Protein? The Effect of Dietary Restriction on Lifespan in Rodents Is Explained by Calories Alone." *Experimental Gerontology* 86 (2016): 28–38.

30. Lee, C., and V. Longo. "Dietary Restriction with and Without Caloric Restriction for Healthy Aging." *F1000Research* 5 (2016).

31. Longo, V. D., and L. Fontana. "Calorie Restriction and Cancer Prevention: Metabolic and Molecular Mechanisms." *Trends in Pharmacological Sciences* 31, no. 2 (2010): 89–98.

32. Fontana, L., et al. "Long-Term Effects of Calorie or Protein Restriction on Serum IGF-1 and IGFBP-3 Concentration in Humans." *Aging Cell* 7, no. 5 (2008): 681–7.

33. Huang, C. H., et al. "EGCG Inhibits Protein Synthesis, Lipogenesis, and Cell Cycle Progression Through Activation of AMPK in p53 Positive and Negative Human Hepatoma Cells." *Molecular Nutrition & Food Research* 53, no. 9 (2009): 1156–65.

34. Pazoki-Toroudi, H., et al. "Targeting mTOR Signaling by Polyphenols: A New Therapeutic Target for Ageing." *Ageing Research Reviews* 31 (2016): 55–66.

35. Chiu, C. T., et al. "Hibiscus Sabdariffa Leaf Polyphenolic Extract Induces Human Melanoma Cell Death, Apoptosis, and Autophagy." *Journal of Food Science* 80, no. 3 (2015): H649–58; Zhang, L., et al. "Polyphenol-Rich Extract of Pimenta Dioica Berries (Allspice) Kills Breast Cancer Cells by Autophagy and Delays Growth of Triple Negative Breast Cancer in Athymic Mice." *Oncotarget* 6, no. 18 (2015): 16379–95; Syed, D. N., et al. "Pomegranate Extracts and Cancer Prevention: Molecular and Cellular Activities." *Anti-Cancer Agents in Medicinal Chemistry* 13, no. 8 (2013): 1149–61.

36. Pazoki-Toroudi, H., et al. "Targeting mTOR Signaling by Polyphenols: A New Therapeutic Target for Ageing." *Ageing Research Reviews* 31 (2016): 55–66; Morselli, E., et al. "Caloric Restriction and Resveratrol Promote Longevity Through the Sirtuin-1-Dependent Induction of Autophagy." *Cell Death Discovery* 1 (2010): e10; Park, S. J., et al. "Resveratrol Ameliorates Aging-Related Metabolic Phenotypes by Inhibiting cAMP Phosphodiesterases." *Cell* 148, no. 3 (2012): 421–33.

37. Zhou, G., et al. "Role of AMP-Activated Protein Kinase in Mechanism of Metformin Action." *Journal of Clinical Investigation* 108, no. 8 (2001): 1167–74.

38. Zi, F., et al. "Metformin and Cancer: An Existing Drug for Cancer Prevention and Therapy." *Oncology Letters* 15, no. 1 (2018): 683–90.

39. Bannister, C. A., et al. "Can People with Type 2 Diabetes Live Longer Than Those Without? A Comparison of Mortality in People Initiated with Metformin or Sulphonylurea Monotherapy and Matched, Non-Diabetic Controls." *Diabetes, Obesity and Metabolism* 16, no. 11 (2014): 1165–73.

40. Rudman, D., et al. "Effects of Human Growth Hormone in Men over 60 Years Old." *New England Journal of Medicine* 323, no. 1 (1990): 1–6.

41. Inagaki, T., et al. "Inhibition of Growth Hormone Signaling by the Fasting-Induced Hormone FGF21." *Cell Metabolism* 8, no. 1 (2008): 77–83.

42. Silberberg, M., and R. Silberberg. "Factors Modifying the Lifespan of Mice." *American Journal of Physiology* 177, no. 1 (1954): 23–6.

43. Grandison, R. C., M. D. Piper, and L. Partridge. "Amino-Acid Imbalance Explains Extension of Lifespan by Dietary Restriction in Drosophila." *Nature* 462, no. 7276 (2009): 1061–4.

44. Kim, E., and K. L. Guan. "RAG GTPases in Nutrient-Mediated TOR Signaling Pathway." *Cell Cycle* 8, no. 7 (2009): 1014–8.

45. McCay, C. M., et al. "The Effect of Retarded Growth upon the Length of Life Span and upon the Ultimate Body Size." *The Journal of Nutrition* 10, no. 1 (1935): 63–79.

46. Liu, K. A., et al. "Leucine Supplementation Differentially Enhances Pancreatic Cancer Growth in Lean and Overweight Mice." *Cancer Metabolism* 2, no. 1 (2014): 6.

47. Huffman, S., and R. J. Jones. "Chronic Effect of Dietary Protein on Hypercholesteremia in the Rat." *Proceedings of the Society for Experimental Biology and Medicine* 93, no. 3 (1956): 519–22.

48. Minor, R. K., et al. "Dietary Interventions to Extend Life Span and Health Span Based on Calorie Restriction." *Journals of Gerontology, Series A: Biological Sciences and Medical Sciences* 65, no. 7 (2010): 695–703.

49. Minor, R. K., et al. "Dietary Interventions to Extend Life Span and Health Span Based on Calorie Restriction." *Journals of Gerontology, Series A: Biological Sciences and Medical Sciences* 65, no. 7 (2010): 695–703; Levine, M. E., et al. "Low Protein Intake Is Associated with a Major Reduction in IGF-1, Cancer, and Overall Mortality in the 65 and Younger but Not Older Population." *Cell Metabolism* 19, no. 3 (2014): 407–17; Solon-Biet, S. M., et al. "The Ratio of Macronutrients, Not Caloric Intake, Dictates Cardiometabolic Health, Aging, and Longevity in Ad Libitum-Fed Mice." *Cell Metabolism* 19, no. 3 (2014): 418–30.

50. Blagosklonny, M. V. "Rapamycin and Quasi-Programmed Aging: Four Years Later." *Cell Cycle* 9, no. 10 (2010): 1859–62.

Chapter 4

1. Levine, M. E., et al. "Low Protein Intake Is Associated with a Major Reduction in IGF-1 Cancer, and Overall Mortality in the 65 and Younger but Not Older Population." *Cell Metabolism* 19, no. 3 (2014): 407–17.

2. Fontana, L., et al. "Long-Term Effects of Calorie or Protein Restriction on Serum IGF-1 and IGFBP-3 Concentration in Humans." *Aging Cell* 7, no. 5 (2008): 681–7.

3. De Bandt, J. P., and L. Cynober. "Therapeutic Use of Branched-Chain Amino Acids in Burn, Trauma, and Sepsis." *Journal of Nutrition* 136, 1 Suppl (2006): 308s–13s.

4. Miller, R. A., et al. "Methionine-Deficient Diet Extends Mouse Lifespan, Slows Immune and Lens Aging, Alters Glucose, T4, IGF-I and Insulin Levels, and Increases Hepatocyte MIF Levels and Stress Resistance." *Aging Cell* 4, no. 3 (2005): 119–25.

5. McCarty, M. F., and J. J. DiNicolantonio. "The Cardiometabolic Benefits of Glycine: Is Glycine an 'Antidote' to Dietary Fructose?" *Open Heart* (2014). 1:e000103. doi:10.1136/openhrt-2014-000103.

6. "Body Fat Calculator." *Active* website. Accessed at *www.active.com/fitness/calculators/bodyfat*.

7. Rosedale, R. "The Good, the Bad, and the Ugly of Protein" (lecture, American Society of Bariatric Physicians (ASBP), October 31, 2006). Accessed at *http://drrosedale.com/resources/pdf/The_good_the_bad_and_the_ugly_of_protein.pdf*.

8. Cuervo, A. M., et al. "Autophagy and Aging: The Importance of Maintaining 'Clean' Cells." *Autophagy* 1, no. 3 (2005): 131–40.

9. Cheng, C. W., et al. "Prolonged Fasting Reduces IGF-1/PKA to Promote Hematopoietic-Stem-Cell-Based Regeneration and Reverse Immunosuppression." *Cell Stem Cell* 14, no. 6 (2014): 810–23.

10. Brandhorst, S., et al. "A Periodic Diet that Mimics Fasting Promotes Multi-System Regeneration, Enhanced Cognitive Performance, and Healthspan." *Cell Metabolism* 22, no. 1 (2015): 86–99.

11. Rosedale, R., E. C. Westman, and J. P. Konhilas. "Clinical Experience of a Diet Designed to Reduce Aging." *Journal of Applied Research* 9, no. 4 (2009): 159–65.

Chapter 5

1. Hancox, D. "The Unstoppable Rise of Veganism: How a Fringe Movement Went Mainstream." *The Guardian*, April 1, 2018. Accessed at *www.theguardian.com/lifeandstyle/2018/apr/01/vegans-are-coming-millennials-health-climate-change-animal-welfare.*

2. Zelman, K. M. "The Power of Plant Protein." United Healthcare. Accessed at *www.uhc.com/health-and-wellness/nutrition/power-of-plant-protein.*

3. "Lacalbumin." *https://en.wikipedia.org/wiki/Lactalbumin.*

4. Bounous, G., and P. Gold. "The Biological Activity of Undenatured Dietary Whey Proteins: Role of Glutathione." *Clinical and Investigative Medicine* 14, no. 4 (1991): 296–309.

5. Bounous, G., G. Batist, and P. Gold. "Whey Proteins in Cancer Prevention." *Cancer Letter* 57, no. 2 (1991): 91–4.

6. Bounous, G., G. Batist, and P. Gold. "Immunoenhancing Property of Dietary Whey Protein in Mice: Role of Glutathione." *Clinical and Investigative Medicine* 12, no. 3 (1989): 154–61.

7. Sekhar, R. V., et al. "Glutathione Synthesis Is Diminished in Patients with Uncontrolled Diabetes and Restored by Dietary Supplementation with Cysteine and Glycine." *Diabetes Care* 34, no. 1 (2011): 162–7.

8. Berk, M., et al. "The Efficacy of N-Acetylcysteine as an Adjunctive Treatment in Bipolar Depression: An Open Label Trial." *Journal of Affective Disorders* 135, no. 1–3 (2011): 389–94.

9. Dean, O., F. Giorlando, and M. Berk. "N-Acetylcysteine in Psychiatry: Current Therapeutic Evidence and Potential Mechanisms of Action." *Journal of Psychiatry & Neuroscience* 36, no. 2 (2011): 78–86.

10. Breitkreutz, R., et al. "Massive Loss of Sulfur in HIV Infection." *AIDS Research and Human Retroviruses* 16, no. 3 (2000): 203–9.

11. Bounous, G., et al. "Whey Proteins as a Food Supplement in HIV-Seropositive Individuals." *Clinical and Investigative Medicine* 16, no. 3 (1993): 204–9.

12. Tse, H. N., et al. "High-Dose N-Acetylcysteine in Stable COPD: The 1-Year, Double-Blind, Randomized, Placebo-Controlled HIACE Study." *Chest* 144, no. 1 (2013): 106–18; De Flora, S., C. Grassi, and L. Carati. "Attenuation of Influenza-Like Symptomatology and Improvement of Cell-Mediated Immunity with Long-Term N-Acetylcysteine Treatment." *European Respiratory Journal* 10, no. 7 (1997): 1535–41.

13. Droge, W. "Oxidative Stress and Ageing: Is Ageing a Cysteine Deficiency Syndrome?" *Philosophical Transactions of the Royal Society B: Biological Sciences* (London) 360, no. 1464 (2005): 2355–72.

14. Op den Kamp, C. M., et al. "Muscle Atrophy in Cachexia: Can Dietary Protein Tip the Balance?" *Current Opinion in Clinical Nutrition & Metabolic Care* 12, no. 6 (2009): 611–6.

15. Marchesini, G., et al. "Nutritional Supplementation with Branched-Chain Amino Acids in Advanced Cirrhosis: A Double-Blind, Randomized Trial." *Gastroenterology* 124, no. 7 (2003): 1792–801.

16. D'Antona, G., et al. "Branched-Chain Amino Acid Supplementation Promotes Survival and Supports Cardiac and Skeletal Muscle Mitochondrial Biogenesis in Middle-Aged Mice." *Cell Metabolism* 12, no. 4 (2010): 362–72.

17. Hoppe, C., et al. "Differential Effects of Casein Versus Whey on Fasting Plasma Levels of Insulin, IGF-1 and IGF-1/IGFBP-3: Results from a Randomized 7-Day Supplementation Study in Prepubertal Boys." *European Journal of Clinical Nutrition* 63, no. 9 (2009): 1076–83.

18. Cheng, Z., et al. "Inhibition of Hepatocellular Carcinoma Development in Hepatitis B Virus Transfected Mice by Low Dietary Casein." *Hepatology* 26, no. 5 (1997): 1351–4.

19. Siri-Tarino, P. W., et al. "Meta-Analysis of Prospective Cohort Studies Evaluating the Association of Saturated Fat with Cardiovascular Disease." *American Journal of Clinical Nutrition* 91, no. 3 (2010): 535–46.

20. Simon, S. "World Health Organization Says Processed Meat Causes Cancer." American Cancer Society, Oct 26, 2015. Accessed at *www.cancer.org/latest-news/world-health-organization-says-processed-meat-causes-cancer.html.*

21. Sugiyama, K., Y. Kushima, and K. Muramatsu. "Effect of Dietary Glycine on Methionine Metabolism in Rats Fed a High-Methionine Diet." *Journal of Nutritional Science and Vitaminology* (Tokyo) 33, no. 3 (1987): 195–205.

22. McCarty, M. F., and J. J. DiNicolantonio. "The Cardiometabolic Benefits of Glycine: Is Glycine an 'Antidote' to Dietary Fructose?" *Open Heart* 1, no. 1 (2014): e000103.

23. Fang, X., et al. "Dietary Magnesium Intake and the Risk of Cardiovascular Disease, Type 2 Diabetes, and All-Cause Mortality: A Dose-Response Meta-Analysis of Prospective Cohort Studies." *BMC Medicine* 14, no. 1 (2016): 210; Adebamowo, S. N., et al. "Association Between Intakes of Magnesium, Potassium, and Calcium and Risk of Stroke: 2 Cohorts of US Women and Updated Meta-Analyses." *American Journal of Clinical Nutrition* 101, no. 6 (2015): 1269–77; Choi, M. K., and Y. J. Bae. "Association of Magnesium Intake with High Blood Pressure in Korean Adults: Korea National Health and Nutrition Examination Survey 2007–2009." *PLoS One* 10, no. 6 (2015): e0130405; and Aburto, N. J., et al. "Effect of Increased Potassium Intake on Cardiovascular Risk Factors and Disease: Systematic Review and Meta-Analyses." *British Medical Journal* 346 (2013): f1378.

24. Song, M., et al. "Association of Animal and Plant Protein Intake with All-Cause and Cause-Specific Mortality." *JAMA Internal Medicine* 176, no. 10 (2016): 1453–63.

25. Key, T. J., et al. "Mortality in British Vegetarians: Review and Preliminary Results from EPIC-Oxford." *American Journal of Clinical Nutrition* 78 (3 Suppl) (2003): 533s–538s.

26. Shinwell, E. D., and R. Gorodischer. "Totally Vegetarian Diets and Infant Nutrition." *Pediatrics* 70, no. 4 (1982): 582–6.

27. McCarty, M. F. "Vegan Proteins May Reduce Risk of Cancer, Obesity, and Cardiovascular Disease by Promoting Increased Glucagon Activity." *Medical Hypotheses* 53, no. 6 (1999): 459–85.

28. Freeman, A. M., et al. "A Clinician's Guide for Trending Cardiovascular Nutrition Controversies: Part II." *Journal of the American College of Cardiology* 72, no. 5 (2018): 553–68.

29. See note 2 above.

30. Mozaffarian, D., et al. "Changes in Diet and Lifestyle and Long-Term Weight Gain in Women and Men." *New England Journal of Medicine* 364, no. 25 (2011): 2392–404.

31. Jaceldo-Siegl, K., et al. "Tree Nuts Are Inversely Associated with Metabolic Syndrome and Obesity: The Adventist Health Study-2." *PLoS One* 9, no. 1 (2014): e85133.

32. Bao, Y., et al. "Association of Nut Consumption with Total and Cause-Specific Mortality." *New England Journal of Medicine* 369, no. 21 (2013): 2001–11.

33. Ibid.

34. Fraser, G. E., and D. J. Shavlik. "Ten Years of Life: Is It a Matter of Choice?" *Archives of Internal Medicine* 161, no. 13 (2001): 1645–52.

35. Rantanen, T., et al. "Midlife Muscle Strength and Human Longevity Up to Age 100 Years: A 44-Year Prospective Study Among a Decedent Cohort." *Age* (Dordrecht, Netherlands) 34, no. 3 (2012): 563–70.

36. Haub, M. D., et al. "Effect of Protein Source on Resistive-Training-Induced Changes in Body Composition and Muscle Size in Older Men." *American Journal of Clinical Nutrition* 76, no. 3 (2002): 511–7.

37. Campbell, W. W., et al. "Effects of an Omnivorous Diet Compared with a Lactoovovegetarian Diet on Resistance-Training-Induced Changes in Body Composition and Skeletal Muscle in Older Men." *American Journal of Clinical Nutrition* 70, no. 6 (1999): 1032–9.

38. Campbell, W. W., et al. "The Recommended Dietary Allowance for Protein May Not Be Adequate for Older People to Maintain Skeletal Muscle." *Journals of Gerontology Series A: Biological Sciences and Medical Sciences* 56, no. 6 (2001): M373–80.

39. Babault, N., et al. "Pea Proteins Oral Supplementation Promotes Muscle Thickness Gains During Resistance Training: A Double-Blind, Randomized, Placebo-Controlled Clinical Trial vs. Whey Protein." *Journal of the International Society of Sports Nutrition* 12, no. 1 (2015): 3.

40. Joy, J. M., et al. "The Effects of 8 Weeks of Whey or Rice Protein Supplementation on Body Composition and Exercise Performance." *Nutrition Journal* 12 (2013): 86.

41. Appel, L. J., et al. "Effects of Protein, Monounsaturated Fat, and Carbohydrate Intake on Blood Pressure and Serum Lipids: Results of the OmniHeart Randomized Trial." *Journal of the American Medical Association* 294, no. 19 (2005): 2455–64.

42. Fung, T. T., et al. "Low-Carbohydrate Diets and All-Cause and Cause-Specific Mortality: Two Cohort Studies." *Annals of Internal Medicine* 153, no. 5 (2010): 289–98.

43. Salvioli, S., et al. "Why Do Centenarians Escape or Postpone Cancer? The Role of IGF-1, Inflammation and p53." *Cancer Immunology, Immunotherapy* 58, no. 12 (2009): 1909–17.

44. Jenkins, D. J., et al. "The Effect of a Plant-Based Low-Carbohydrate ('Eco-Atkins') Diet on Body Weight and Blood Lipid Concentrations in Hyperlipidemic Subjects." *Archives of Internal Medicine* 169, no. 11 (2009): 1046–54.

45. Kiefte-de Jong, J. C., et al. "Diet-Dependent Acid Load and Type 2 Diabetes: Pooled Results from Three Prospective Cohort Studies." *Diabetologia* 60, no. 2 (2017): 270–9.

46. Frassetto, L., et al. "Diet, Evolution and Aging—the Pathophysiologic Effects of the Post-Agricultural Inversion of the Potassium-to-Sodium and Base-to-Chloride Ratios in the Human Diet." *European Journal of Nutrition* 40, no. 5 (2001): 200–13.

47. Frassetto, L. A., et al. "Worldwide Incidence of Hip Fracture in Elderly Women: Relation to Consumption of Animal and Vegetable Foods." *Journal of Gerontology Series A: Biological Sciences Med Sci* 55, no. 10 (2000): M585–92.

48. See notes 46 and 47 above.

49. Jackson, R. D., et al. "Calcium Plus Vitamin D Supplementation and the Risk of Fractures." *New England Journal of Medicine* 354, no. 7 (2006): 669–83.

50. Reddy, S. T., et al. "Effect of Low-Carbohydrate High-Protein Diets on Acid-Base Balance, Stone-Forming Propensity, and Calcium Metabolism." *American Journal of Kidney Disease* 40, no. 2 (2002): 265–74.

51. Sebastian, A., et al. "Improved Mineral Balance and Skeletal Metabolism in Postmenopausal Women Treated with Potassium Bicarbonate." *New England Journal of Medicine* 330, no. 25 (1994): 1776–81; and Goraya, N., et al. "Dietary Acid Reduction with Fruits and Vegetables or Bicarbonate Attenuates Kidney Injury in Patients with a Moderately Reduced Glomerular Filtration Rate Due to Hypertensive Nephropathy." *Kidney International* 81, no. 1 (2012): 86–93.

Chapter 6

1. Food and Nutrition Board, Institute of Medicine of the National Academies. "Dietary Reference Intakes for Energy, Carbohydrate, Fiber, Fat, Fatty Acids, Cholesterol, Protein, and Amino Acids." National Academies Press (2005). Accessed at *www.nap.edu/read/10490/chapter/1*.

2. Humayun, M. A., et al. "Reevaluation of the Protein Requirement in Young Men with the Indicator Amino Acid Oxidation Technique." *American Journal of Clinical Nutrition* 86, no. 4 (2007): 995–1002.

3. Jackson, A. A., et al. "Synthesis of Erythrocyte Glutathione in Healthy Adults Consuming the Safe Amount of Dietary Protein." *American Journal of Clinical Nutrition* 80, no. 1 (2004): 101–7.

4. Zelman, K. "The Power of Plant Protein." United HealthCare Services Inc. Accessed at *www.uhc.com/health-and-wellness/nutrition/power-of-plant-protein*.

5. Dupont, C. "Protein Requirements During the First Year of Life." *American Journal of Clinical Nutrition* 77, no. 6 (2003): 1544s–9s.

6. Gartner, L. M., et al. "Breastfeeding and the Use of Human Milk." *Pediatrics* 115, no. 2 (2005): 496–506.

7. Stephens, T. V., et al. "Protein Requirements of Healthy Pregnant Women During Early and Late Gestation Are Higher Than Current Recommendations." *Journal of Nutrition* 145, no. 1 (2015): 73–8.

8. Kortebein, P., et al. "Effect of 10 Days of Bed Rest on Skeletal Muscle in Healthy Older Adults." *Journal of the American Medical Association* 297, no. 16 (2007): 1772–4.

9. Bauer, J., et al. "Evidence-Based Recommendations for Optimal Dietary Protein Intake in Older People: A Position Paper from the PROT-AGE Study Group." *Journal of the American Medical Directors Association* 14, no. 8 (2013): 542–59.

10. Alexander, J. W., et al. "The Importance of Lipid Type in the Diet After Burn Injury." *Annals of Surgery* 204, no. 1 (1986): 1–8; Berbert, A. A., et al. "Supplementation of Fish Oil and Olive Oil in Patients with Rheumatoid Arthritis." *Nutrition* 21, no. 2 (2005): 131–6; Murphy, R. A., et al. "Nutritional Intervention with Fish Oil Provides a Benefit Over Standard of Care for Weight and Skeletal Muscle Mass in Patients with Nonsmall Cell Lung Cancer Receiving Chemotherapy." *Cancer* 117, no. 8 (2011): 1775–82; Rodacki, C. L., et al. "Fish-Oil Supplementation Enhances the Effects of Strength Training in Elderly Women." *American Journal of Clinical Nutrition* 95, no. 2 (2012): 428–36; and Ryan, A. M., et al. "Enteral Nutrition Enriched with Eicosapentaenoic Acid (EPA) Preserves Lean Body Mass Following Esophageal Cancer Surgery: Results of a Double-Blinded Randomized Controlled Trial." *Annals of Surgery* 249, no. 3 (2009): 355–63.

11. McWhirter, J., and C. R. Pennington. "Incidence and Recognition of Malnutrition in Hospital." *British Medical Journal* 308, no. 6934 (1994): 945–8.

12. Centers for Disease Control and Prevention. "Healthcare-Associated Infections." Accessed at *www.cdc.gov/HAI/surveillance/*.

13. Aquilani, R., et al. "Effects of Oral Amino Acid Supplementation on Long-Term-Care-Acquired Infections in Elderly Patients." *Archives of Gerontology and Geriatrics* 52, no. 3 (2011): e123–8.

14. Brown, R. O., et al. "Comparison of Specialized and Standard Enteral Formulas in Trauma Patients." *Pharmacotherapy* 14, no. 3 (1994): 314–20.

15. Paddon-Jones, D., et al. "Essential Amino Acid and Carbohydrate Supplementation Ameliorates Muscle Protein Loss in Humans During 28 Days Bedrest." *Journal of Clinical Endocrinology Metabolism* 89, no. 9 (2004): 4351–8.

16. Stokes, T., et al. "Recent Perspectives Regarding the Role of Dietary Protein for the Promotion of Muscle Hypertrophy with Resistance Exercise Training." *Nutrients* 10, no. 2 (2018).

17. Ibid.

18. Ibid.

19. Ibid.

20. Ibid.

21. Ibid.

22. Macnaughton, L. S., et al. "The Response of Muscle Protein Synthesis Following Whole-Body Resistance Exercise Is Greater Following 40 g Than 20 g of Ingested Whey Protein." *Physiology Report* 4, no. 15 (2016).

23. See note 16 above.

24. Ibid.

25. Lemon, P. W. "Beyond the Zone: Protein Needs of Active Individuals." *Journal of the American College of Nutrition* 19, 5 Suppl (2000): 513s–21s.

26. See note 16 above.

27. Ibid.

28. Li, P., and G. Wu. "Roles of Dietary Glycine, Proline, and Hydroxyproline in Collagen Synthesis and Animal Growth." *Amino Acids* 50, no. 1 (2018): 29–38; Melendez-Hevia, E., et al. "A Weak Link in Metabolism: The Metabolic Capacity for Glycine Biosynthesis Does Not Satisfy the Need for Collagen Synthesis." *Journal of Bioscience* 34, no. 6 (2009): 853–72.

29. McCarty, M. F., and J. J. DiNicolantonio. "The Cardiometabolic Benefits of Glycine: Is Glycine an 'Antidote' to Dietary Fructose?" *Open Heart* 1, no. 1 (2014): e000103.

30. See note 16 above.

31. Ibid.

32. Tarnopolsky, M. A., J. D. MacDougall, and S. A. Atkinson. "Influence of Protein Intake and Training Status on Nitrogen Balance and Lean Body Mass." *Journal of Applied Physiology* (1985) 64, no. 1 (1988): 187–93.

33. Ibid.

34. Kingsbury, K. J., L. Kay, and M. Hjelm. "Contrasting Plasma Free Amino Acid Patterns in Elite Athletes: Association with Fatigue and Infection." *British Journal of Sports Medicine* 32, no. 1 (1998): 25–32; discussion 32–3.

35. Rantanen, T., et al. "Midlife Muscle Strength and Human Longevity Up to Age 100 Years: A 44-Year Prospective Study Among a Decedent Cohort." *Age* (Dordr) 34, no. 3 (2012): 563–70.

36. Layman, D. K., et al., "A Reduced Ratio of Dietary Carbohydrate to Protein Improves Body Composition and Blood Lipid Profiles During Weight Loss in Adult Women." *Journal of Nutrition* 133, no. 2 (2003): 411–7.

37. Frestedt, J. L., et al. "A Whey-Protein Supplement Increases Fat Loss and Spares Lean Muscle in Obese Subjects: A Randomized Human Clinical Study." *Nutrition & Metabolism* (London) 5 (2008): 8.

38. Demling, R. H., and L. DeSanti. "Effect of a Hypocaloric Diet, Increased Protein Intake and Resistance Training on Lean Mass Gains and Fat Mass Loss in Overweight Police Officers." *Annals of Nutrition and Metabolism* 44, no. 1 (2000): 21–9.

39. Simpson, S. J., and D. Raubenheimer. "Obesity: The Protein Leverage Hypothesis." *Obesity Review* 6, no. 2 (2005): 133–42.

40. Leaf, A. "How Much Protein Do You Need Per Day?" Examine.com. Accessed at *https://examine.com/nutrition/how-much-protein-do-i-need/*.

41. Kopple, J. D. "National Kidney Foundation K/DOQI Clinical Practice Guidelines for Nutrition in Chronic Renal Failure." *American Journal of Kidney Disease* 37, 1 Suppl 2 (2001): S66–70.

42. Ibid.

43. English, K. L., and D. Paddon-Jones. "Protecting Muscle Mass and Function in Older Adults During Bed Rest." *Current Opinion in Clinical Nutrition & Metabolic Care* 13, no. 1 (2010): 34–9.

44. Patel, K. "How Much Protein Do You Need After Exercise?" Examine.com. Accessed at *https://examine.com/nutrition/second-look-at-protein-quantity-after-exercise/*.

Chapter 7

1. Nuttall, F. Q., and M. C. Gannon. "Metabolic Response to Dietary Protein in People with and Without Diabetes." *Diabetes, Nutrition and Metabolism* 4 (1991): 71–88.

2. Cahill, G. F., Jr. "Fuel Metabolism in Starvation." *Annual Review of Nutrition* 26 (2006): 1–22.

3. Hall, K. D. *Comparative Physiology of Fasting, Starvation, and Food Limitation*, ed. Marshall McCue. Berlin: Springer, 2012. Accessed at *www.cussp.org/sites/default/files/Hall%20Slides.pdf.*

4. Bhutani, S., et al. "Improvements in Coronary Heart Disease Risk Indicators by Alternate-Day Fasting Involve Adipose Tissue Modulations." *Obesity* (Silver Spring), 18, no. 11 (2010): 2152–9.

5. Catenacci, V. A., et al. "A Randomized Pilot Study Comparing Zero-Calorie Alternate-Day Fasting to Daily Caloric Restriction in Adults with Obesity." *Obesity* (Silver Spring) 24, no. 9 (2016): 1874–83.

6. Zauner, C., et al. "Resting Energy Expenditure in Short-Term Starvation Is Increased as a Result of an Increase in Serum Norepinephrine." *American Journal of Clinical Nutrition* 71, no. 6 (2000): 1511–5.

7. Ho, K. Y., et al. "Fasting Enhances Growth Hormone Secretion and Amplifies the Complex Rhythms of Growth Hormone Secretion in Man." *Journal of Clinical Investigation* 81, no. 4 (1988): 968–75.

8. Cahill, G. F., Jr. "President's Address. Starvation." *Transactions of the American Clinical and Climatological Association* 94 (1983): 1–21.

9. Henry, C. J. K., et al. "Differences in Fat, Carbohydrate, and Protein Metabolism Between Lean and Obese Subjects Undergoing Total Starvation." *Obesity Research* 7, no. 6 (1999): 597–604.

10. See note 9 above.

11. Ibid.

Chapter 8

1. Di Castelnuovo, A., et al. "Consumption of Cocoa, Tea and Coffee and Risk of Cardiovascular Disease." *European Journal of Internal Medicine* 23, no. 1 (2012): 15–25.

2. Huxley, R. R., and H. A. Neil. "The Relation Between Dietary Flavonol Intake and Coronary Heart Disease Mortality: A Meta-Analysis of Prospective Cohort Studies." *European Journal of Clinical Nutrition* 57, no. 8 (2003): 904–8.

3. Hodgson, J. M., and K. D. Croft. "Tea Flavonoids and Cardiovascular Health." *Molecular Aspects of Medicine* 31, no. 6 (2010): 495–502.

4. de Koning Gans, J. M., et al. "Tea and Coffee Consumption and Cardiovascular Morbidity and Mortality." *Arteriosclerosis, Thrombosis, and Vascular Biology* 30, no. 8 (2010): 1665–71.

5. Peters, U., C. Poole, and L. Arab. "Does Tea Affect Cardiovascular Disease? A Meta-Analysis." *American Journal of Epidemiology* 154, no. 6 (2001): 495–503.

6. Geleijnse, J. M., et al. "Inverse Association of Tea and Flavonoid Intakes with Incident Myocardial Infarction: The Rotterdam Study." *American Journal of Clinical Nutrition* 75, no. 5 (2002): 880–6.

7. Pang, J., et al. "Green Tea Consumption and Risk of Cardiovascular and Ischemic Related Diseases: A Meta-Analysis." *International Journal of Cardiology* 202 (2012): 967–74.

8. Kuriyama, S., et al. "Green Tea Consumption and Mortality Due to Cardiovascular Disease, Cancer, and All Causes in Japan: The Ohsaki Study." *JAMA* 296, no. 10 (2006): 1255–65.

9. Hertog, M. G., et al. "Antioxidant Flavonols and Ischemic Heart Disease in a Welsh Population of Men: The Caerphilly Study." *American Journal of Clinical Nutrition* 65, no. 5 (1997): 1489–94.

10. Serafini, M., A. Ghiselli, and A. Ferro-Luzzi. "In Vivo Antioxidant Effect of Green and Black Tea in Man." *European Journal of Clinical Nutrition* 50, no. 1 (1996): 28–32.

11. Arab, L., W. Liu, and D. Elashoff. "Green and Black Tea Consumption and Risk of Stroke: A Meta-Analysis." *Stroke* 40, no. 5 (2009): 1786–92.

12. Chen, I. J., et al. "Therapeutic Effect of High-Dose Green Tea Extract on Weight Reduction: A Randomized, Double-Blind, Placebo-Controlled Clinical Trial." *Clinical Nutrition* 35, no. 3 (2016): 592–9.

13. Hursel, R., W. Viechtbauer, and M. S. Westerterp-Plantenga. "The Effects of Green Tea on Weight Loss and Weight Maintenance: A Meta-Analysis." *International Journal of Obesity* (London) 33, no. 9 (2009): 956–61.

14. Rudelle, S., et al. "Effect of a Thermogenic Beverage on 24-Hour Energy Metabolism in Humans." *Obesity* (Silver Spring) 15, no. 2 (2007): 349–55.

15. Dulloo, A. G., et al. "Efficacy of a Green Tea Extract Rich in Catechin Polyphenols and Caffeine in Increasing 24-H Energy Expenditure and Fat Oxidation in Humans." *American Journal of Clinical Nutrition* 70, no. 6 (1999): 1040–5; Hursel, R., et al. "The Effects of Catechin Rich Teas and Caffeine on Energy Expenditure and Fat Oxidation: A Meta-Analysis." *Obesity Review* 12, no. 7 (2011): 573–81.

16. Jurgens, T. M., et al. "Green Tea for Weight Loss and Weight Maintenance in Overweight or Obese Adults." *Cochrane Database of Systematic Reviews* 12 (2012): Cd008650.

17. Rumpler, W., et al. "Oolong Tea Increases Metabolic Rate and Fat Oxidation in Men." *Journal of Nutrition* 131, no. 11 (2001): 2848–52.

18. Thielecke, F., and M. Boschmann. "The Potential Role of Green Tea Catechins in the Prevention of the Metabolic Syndrome - A Review." *Phytochemistry* 70, no. 1 (2009): 11–24.

19. Nagao, T., et al. "A Catechin-Rich Beverage Improves Obesity and Blood Glucose Control in Patients with Type 2 Diabetes." *Obesity* (Silver Spring) 17, no. 2 (2009): 310–7.

20. Iso, H., et al. "The Relationship Between Green Tea and Total Caffeine Intake and Risk for Self-Reported Type 2 Diabetes Among Japanese Adults." *Annals of Internal Medicine* 144, no. 8 (2006): 554–62.

21. Panagiotakos, D. B., et al. "Long-Term Tea Intake Is Associated with Reduced Prevalence of (Type 2) Diabetes Mellitus Among Elderly People from Mediterranean Islands: MEDIS Epidemiological Study." *Yonsei Medical Journal* 50, no. 1 (2009): 31–8.

22. See note 13 above.

23. Stensvold, I., et al. "Tea Consumption. Relationship to Cholesterol, Blood Pressure, and Coronary and Total Mortality." *Preventive Medicine* 21, no. 4 (1992): 546–53.

24. Hodgson, J. M. "Effects of Tea and Tea Flavonoids on Endothelial Function and Blood Pressure: A Brief Review." *Clinical and Experimental Pharmacology and Physiology* 33, no. 9 (2006): 838–41.

25. Yang, Y. C., et al. "The Protective Effect of Habitual Tea Consumption on Hypertension." *Archives of Internal Medicine* 164, no. 14 (2004): 1534–40.

26. Bogdanski, P., et al. "Green Tea Extract Reduces Blood Pressure, Inflammatory Biomarkers, and Oxidative Stress and Improves Parameters Associated with Insulin Resistance in Obese, Hypertensive Patients." *Nutrition Research* 32, no. 6 (2012): 421–7.

27. "Tea and Cancer Prevention." National Cancer Institute. November 17, 2010. Accessed at *www.cancer.gov/about-cancer/causes-prevention/risk/diet/tea-fact-sheet*.

28. Wu, A. H., et al. "Tea Intake, COMT Genotype, and Breast Cancer in Asian-American Women." *Cancer Research* 63, no. 21 (2003): 7526–9.

29. Fujiki, H., et al., "Cancer Prevention with Green Tea and Its Principal Constituent, EGCG: From Early Investigations to Current Focus on Human Cancer Stem Cells." *Molecules and Cells* 41, no. 2 (2018): 73–82.

Chapter 9

1. Fragopoulou, E., C. Demopoulos, and S. Antonopoulou. "Lipid Minor Constituents in Wines. A Biochemical Approach in the French Paradox." *International Journal of Wine Research* 1 (2009): 131–43.

2. Nagahori, Z. "Credibility of the Ages of Centenarians in Hunza, a Longevity Village in Pakistan." *Asian Medical Journal* 25, no. 6 (1982): 405–31.

3. Ibid.

4. *Hippocratic Writings*, ed. G. E. R. Lloyd. London: Penguin, 2005. Accessed at *https://books.google.com/books?id=pg-trVeUovEC&lpg=PT93&pg=PT352#v=onepage&q&f=false*.

5. See note 1 above.

6. Osborn, D. "Drink to Your Health!" Accessed at *www.greekmedicine.net/therapies/Drink_to_Your Health.html*.

7. Jouanna, J. *Greek Medicine from Hippocrates to Galen*. Leiden, The Netherlands: Brill, 2012: 173–93.

8. Goldfinger, T. M. "Beyond the French Paradox: The Impact of Moderate Beverage Alcohol and Wine Consumption in the Prevention of Cardiovascular Disease." *Cardiology Clinics* 21, no. 3 (2003): 449–57.

9. Ibid.

10. Galinski, C. N., J. I. Zwicker, and D. R. Kennedy. "Revisiting the Mechanistic Basis of the French Paradox: Red Wine Inhibits the Activity of Protein Disulfide Isomerase In Vitro." *Thrombosis Research* 137 (2016): 169–73.

11. See note 1 above.

12. Ibid.

13. St Leger, A. S., A. L. Cochrane, and F. Moore. "Factors Associated with Cardiac Mortality in Developed Countries with Particular Reference to the Consumption of Wine." *Lancet* 1, no. 8124 (1979): 1017–20.

14. Gronbaek, M., et al. "Mortality Associated with Moderate Intakes of Wine, Beer, or Spirits." *The BMJ* 310, no. 6988 (1995): 1165–9.

15. Renaud, S. C., et al. "Wine, Beer, and Mortality in Middle-Aged Men from Eastern France." *Archives of Internal Medicine* 159, no. 16 (1999): 1865–70.

16. Yuan, J. M., et al. "Follow Up Study of Moderate Alcohol Intake and Mortality Among Middle Aged Men in Shanghai, China." *The BMJ* 1314, no. 7073 (1997): 18–23.

17. Thun, M. J., et al. "Alcohol Consumption and Mortality Among Middle-Aged and Elderly U.S. Adults." *New England Journal of Medicine* 337, no. 24 (1997): 1705–14.

18. Blackhurst, D. M., and A. D. Marais. "Alcohol—Foe or Friend?" *South African Medical Journal* 95, no. 9 (2005): 648–54.

19. Andreasson, S., P. Allebeck, and A. Romelsjo. "Alcohol and Mortality Among Young Men: Longitudinal Study of Swedish Conscripts." *British Medical Journal (Clinical Research Edition)* 296, no. 6628 (1988): 1021–5.

20. Djousse, L., et al. "Alcohol Consumption and Risk of Cardiovascular Disease and Death in Women: Potential Mediating Mechanisms." *Circulation* 2120, no. 3 (2009): 237–44.

21. Streppel, M. T., et al. "Long-Term Wine Consumption Is Related to Cardiovascular Mortality and Life Expectancy Independently of Moderate Alcohol Intake: The Zutphen Study." *Journal of Epidemiology and Community Health* 63, no. 7 (2009): 534–40.

22. Haseeb, S., B. Alexander, and A. Baranchuk. "Wine and Cardiovascular Health: A Comprehensive Review." *Circulation* 136, no. 15 (2017): 1434–48.

23. Covas, M. I., et al. "Wine and Oxidative Stress: Up-to-Date Evidence of the Effects of Moderate Wine Consumption on Oxidative Damage in Humans." *Atherosclerosis* 208, no. 2 (2010): 297–304.

24. See notes 1 and 10 above.

25. Biagi, M., and A. A. Bertelli. "Wine, Alcohol and Pills: What Future for the French Paradox?" *Life Sciences* 131 (2015): 19–22.

26. Sato, M., N. Maulik, and D. K. Das. "Cardioprotection with Alcohol: Role of Both Alcohol and Polyphenolic Antioxidants." *Annals of the New York Academy of Sciences* 957 (2002): 122–35; Guiraud, A., et al. "Cardioprotective Effect of Chronic Low Dose Ethanol Drinking: Insights into the Concept of Ethanol Preconditioning." *Journal of Molecular and Cellular Cardiology* 36, no. 4 (2004): 561–6; Marfella, R., et al. "Effect of Moderate Red Wine Intake on Cardiac Prognosis

After Recent Acute Myocardial Infarction of Subjects with Type 2 Diabetes Mellitus." *Diabetic Medicine* 23, no. 9 (2006): 974–81.

27. Karatzi, K. N., et al. "Red Wine Acutely Induces Favorable Effects on Wave Reflections and Central Pressures in Coronary Artery Disease Patients." *American Journal of Hypertension* 18, no. 9 Pt 1 (2005): 1161–7; Stranges, S., et al. "Relationship of Alcohol Drinking Pattern to Risk of Hypertension: A Population-Based Study." *Hypertension* 44, no. 6 (2004): 813–9.

28. Xin, X., et al. "Effects of Alcohol Reduction on Blood Pressure: A Meta-Analysis of Randomized Controlled Trials." *Hypertension* 38, no. 5 (2001): 1112–7.

29. Lazarus, R., D. Sparrow, and S. T. Weiss. "Alcohol Intake and Insulin Levels. The Normative Aging Study." *American Journal of Epidemiology* 145, no. 10 (1997): 909–16.

30. Koppes, L. L., et al. "Moderate Alcohol Consumption Lowers the Risk of Type 2 Diabetes: A Meta-Analysis of Prospective Observational Studies." *Diabetes Care* 28, no. 3 (2005): 719–25.

31. Shai, I., et al. "Glycemic Effects of Moderate Alcohol Intake Among Patients with Type 2 Diabetes: A Multicenter, Randomized, Clinical Intervention Trial." *Diabetes Care* 30, no. 12 (2007): 3011–6.

32. Corrao, G., et al. "Alcohol and Coronary Heart Disease: A Meta-Analysis." *Addiction* 95, no. 10 (2000): 1505–23.

33. Szmitko, P. E., and S. Verma. "Antiatherogenic Potential of Red Wine: Clinician Update." *American Journal of Physiology-Heart and Circulatory Physiology* 288, no. 5 (2005): H2023–30.

34. Shai, I., et al. "Glycemic Effects of Moderate Alcohol Intake Among Patients with Type 2 Diabetes: A Multicenter, Randomized, Clinical Intervention Trial." *Diabetes Care* 30, no. 12 (2007): 3011–6; Brand-Miller, J. C., et al. "Effect of Alcoholic Beverages on Postprandial Glycemia and Insulinemia in Lean, Young, Healthy Adults." *American Journal of Clinical Nutrition* 85, no. 6 (2007): 1545–51.

35. "The History of Coffee." *NCA* website. Accessed at *www.ncausa.org/about-coffee/history-of-coffee.*

36. Ibid.

37. O'Keefe, J. H., et al. "Effects of Habitual Coffee Consumption on Cardiometabolic Disease, Cardiovascular Health, and All-Cause Mortality." *Journal of the American College of Cardiology* 62, no. 12 (2013): 1043–51.

38. van Dam, R. M., and F. B. Hu. "Coffee Consumption and Risk of Type 2 Diabetes: A Systematic Review." *JAMA* 294, no. 1 (2005): 97–104.

39. Ohnaka, K., et al. "Effects of 16-Week Consumption of Caffeinated and Decaffeinated Instant Coffee on Glucose Metabolism in a Randomized Controlled Trial." *Journal of Nutrition and Metabolism* 2012 (2012): 207426.

40. Ibid.

41. Keijzers, G. B., et al. "Caffeine Can Decrease Insulin Sensitivity in Humans." *Diabetes Care* 25, no. 2 (2002): 364–9.

42. Ding, M., et al. "Caffeinated and Decaffeinated Coffee Consumption and Risk of Type 2 Diabetes: A Systematic Review and a Dose-Response Meta-Analysis." *Diabetes Care* 37, no. 2 (2014): 569–86; Huxley, R., et al. "Coffee, Decaffeinated Coffee, and Tea Consumption in Relation to Incident Type 2 Diabetes Mellitus: A Systematic Review with Meta-Analysis." *Archives of Internal Medicine* 169, no. 22 (2009): 2053–63.

43. Iso, H., et al. "The Relationship Between Green Tea and Total Caffeine Intake and Risk for Self-Reported Type 2 Diabetes Among Japanese Adults." *Annals of Internal Medicine* 144, no. 8 (2006): 554–62.

44. DiNicolantonio, J. J., S. C. Lucan, and J. H. O'Keefe. "Is Coffee Harmful? If Looking for Longevity, Say Yes to the Coffee, No to the Sugar." *Mayo Clinic Proceedings* 89, no. 4 (2014): 576–7.

45. Wedick, N. M., et al. "Effects of Caffeinated and Decaffeinated Coffee on Biological Risk Factors for Type 2 Diabetes: A Randomized Controlled Trial." *Nutrition Journal* 10 (2011): 93.

46. O'Keefe, J. H., J. J. DiNicolantonio, and C. J. Lavie. "Coffee for Cardioprotection and Longevity." *Progress in Cardiovascular Disease* 61, no. 1 (2018).

47. de Koning Gans, J. M., et al. "Tea and Coffee Consumption and Cardiovascular Morbidity and Mortality." *Arteriosclerosis, Thrombosis, and Vascular Biology* 30, no. 8 (2010): 1665–71.

48. Poole, R., et al. "Coffee Consumption and Health: Umbrella Review of Meta-Analyses of Multiple Health Outcomes." *The BMJ* 359 (2017): j5024.

49. Gunter, M. J., et al. " Coffee Drinking and Mortality in 10 European Countries: A Multinational Cohort Study." *Annals of Internal Medicine* 167, no. 4 (2017): 236–47.

50. Ding, M., et al. "Association of Coffee Consumption with Total and Cause-Specific Mortality in 3 Large Prospective Cohorts." *Circulation* 132, no. 24 (2015): 2305–15.

51. Renouf, M., et al. "Plasma Appearance and Correlation Between Coffee and Green Tea Metabolites in Human Subjects." *British Journal of Nutrition* 104, no. 11 (2010): 1635–40.

52. Ojha, S., et al. "Neuroprotective Potential of Ferulic Acid in the Rotenone Model of Parkinson's Disease." *Drug Design, Development and Therapy* (2015): 5499–510; Madeira, M. H., et al. "Having a Coffee Break: The Impact of Caffeine Consumption on Microglia-Mediated Inflammation in Neurodegenerative Diseases." *Mediators of Inflammation* 2017 (2017): 4761081.

53. Ma, Z. C., et al. "Ferulic Acid Induces Heme Oxygenase-1 via Activation of ERK and Nrf2." *Drug Discoveries & Therapeutics* 5, no. 6 (2011): 299–305.

54. Graf, E. "Antioxidant Potential of Ferulic Acid." *Free Radical Biology & Medicine* 13, no. 4 (1992): 435–48.

55. Ren, Z., et al. "Ferulic Acid Exerts Neuroprotective Effects Against Cerebral Ischemia/Reperfusion-Induced Injury via Antioxidant and Anti-Apoptotic Mechanisms In Vitro and In Vivo." *International Journal of Molecular Medicine* 40, no. 5 (2017): 1444–56.

56. Zhao, J., et al. "Ferulic Acid Enhances the Vasorelaxant Effect of Epigallocatechin Gallate in Tumor Necrosis Factor-Alpha-Induced Inflammatory Rat Aorta." *The Journal of Nutritional Biochemistry* 25, no. 7 (2014): 807–14; Zhao, J., et al. "Ferulic Acid Enhances Nitric Oxide Production Through Up-Regulation of Argininosuccinate Synthase in Inflammatory Human Endothelial Cells." *Life Sciences* 145 (2016): 224–32.

57. O'Keefe, J. H., et al. "Effects of Habitual Coffee Consumption on Cardiometabolic Disease, Cardiovascular Health, and All-Cause Mortality." *Journal of the American College of Cardiology* 62, no. 12 (2013): 1043–51; Neuhauser, B., et al. "Coffee Consumption and Total Body Water Homeostasis as Measured by Fluid Balance and Bioelectrical Impedance Analysis." *Annals of Nutrition and Metabolism* 41, no. 1 (1997): 29–36.

58. Massey, L. K., and S. J. Whiting. "Caffeine, Urinary Calcium, Calcium Metabolism and Bone." *Journal of Nutrition* 123, no. 9 (1993): 1611–4.

59. Passmore, A. P., G. B. Kondowe, and G. D. Johnston. "Renal and Cardiovascular Effects of Caffeine: A Dose-Response Study." *Clinical Science* (Lond) 72, no. 6 (1987): 749–56.

Chapter 10

1. Meneely, G. R., and H. D. Battarbee. "High Sodium-Low Potassium Environment and Hypertension. *American Journal of Cardiology* 38, no. 6 (1976): 768–85.

2. Dahl, L. K. "Possible Role of Salt Intake in the Development of Essential Hypertension. 1960." *International Journal of Epidemiology* 34, no. 5 (2005): 967–72; discussion 972–4, 975–8.

3. Dahl, L. K. "Salt in Processed Baby Foods." *American Journal of Clinical Nutrition* 21, no. 8 (1968): 787–92.

4. See note 2 above.

5. DiNicolantonio, J. J., and S. C. Lucan. "The Wrong White Crystals: Not Salt but Sugar as Aetiological in Hypertension and Cardiometabolic Disease." *Open Heart* 1 (2014): doi:10.1136/openhrt-2014-000167; DiNicolantonio, J. J., S. C. Lucan, and J. H. O'Keefe. "An Unsavory Truth: Sugar, More Than Salt, Predisposes to Hypertension and Chronic Disease." *American Journal of Cardiology* 114, no. 7 (2014): 1126–8.

6. DiNicolantonio, J. J. *The Salt Fix: Why the Experts Got It All Wrong—and How Eating More Might Save Your Life*. New York: Harmony (2017).

7. Satin, M. "The Salt Debate—Far More Salacious Than Salubrious." *Blood Purification* 39, no. 1–3 (2015): 11–5.

8. Gleibermann, L. "Blood Pressure and Dietary Salt in Human Populations." *Ecology of Food and Nutrition* 2, no. 2 (1973): 143–56.

9. See note 6 above.

10. Powles, J., et al. "Global, Regional and National Sodium Intakes in 1990 and 2010: A Systematic Analysis of 24 h Urinary Sodium Excretion and Dietary Surveys Worldwide." *BMJ Open* 3, no. 12 (2013). Accessed at *https://bmjopen.bmj.com/content/3/12/e003733*.

11. See note 8 above.

12. Ibid.

13. See note 7 above.

14. Alderman, M. H., H. Cohen, and S. Madhavan. "Dietary Sodium Intake and Mortality: The National Health and Nutrition Examination Survey (NHANES I)." *The Lancet* 351, no. 9105 (1998): 781–5.

15. Ibid.

16. McGuire, S., Institute of Medicine. 2013. *Sodium Intake in Populations: Assessment of Evidence*. Washington, DC: The National Academies Press, 2013.

17. Ibid.

18. See note 1 above.

19. "AACC Members Agree on Definition of Whole Grain." Accessed at *www.aaccnet.org/initiatives/definitions/Documents/WholeGrains/wgflyer.pdf*.

20. "Collagen." *https://en.wikipedia.org/wiki/Collagen*.

21. Sharp, R. L. "Role of Sodium in Fluid Homeostasis with Exercise." *The Journal of the American College of Nutrition* 25, no. 3 Suppl (2006): 231s–239s.

22. See note 5 above.

23. Stolarz-Skrzypek, K., et al. "Fatal and Nonfatal Outcomes, Incidence of Hypertension, and Blood Pressure Changes in Relation to Urinary Sodium Excretion." *JAMA* 30, no. 17 (2011): 1777–85.

24. Feldman, R. D., and N. D. Schmidt. "Moderate Dietary Salt Restriction Increases Vascular and Systemic Insulin Resistance." *American Journal of Hypertension* 12, no. 6 (1999): 643–7.

25. Patel, S. M., et al. "Dietary Sodium Reduction Does Not Affect Circulating Glucose Concentrations in Fasting Children or Adults: Findings from a Systematic Review and Meta-Analysis." *Journal of Nutrition* 145, no. 3 (2015): 505–13.

26. Graudal, N. A., A. M. Galloe, and P. Garred. "Effects of Sodium Restriction on Blood Pressure, Renin, Aldosterone, Catecholamines, Cholesterols, and Triglyceride: A Meta-Analysis." *JAMA* 279, no. 17 (1998): 1383–91.

27. See note 6 above.

28. O'Donnell, M., et al. "Urinary Sodium and Potassium Excretion, Mortality, and Cardiovascular Events." *New England Journal of Medicine* 371, no. 7 (2014): 612–23.

29. Graudal, N., et al. "Compared with Usual Sodium Intake, Low- and Excessive-Sodium Diets Are Associated with Increased Mortality: A Meta-Analysis." *American Journal of Hypertension* 27, no. 9 (2014): 1129–37.

30. Folkow, B. "Salt and Blood Pressure—Centenarian Bone of Contention." *Lakartidningen* 100, no. 40 (2003): 3142–7.

31. Liedtke, W. B., et al. "Relation of Addiction Genes to Hypothalamic Gene Changes Subserving Genesis and Gratification of a Classic Instinct, Sodium Appetite." *Proceedings of the National Academy of Sciences of the United States of America* 108, no. 30 (2011): 12509–14.

32. Denton, D. A., M. J. McKinley, and R. S. Weisinger. "Hypothalamic Integration of Body Fluid Regulation." *Proceedings of the National Academy of Sciences of the United States of America* 93, no. 14 (1996): 7397–404.

33. Adler, A. J., et al. "Reduced Dietary Salt for the Prevention of Cardiovascular Disease." *Cochrane Database Systematic Reviews* 12 (2014): Cd009217.

34. Kelly, J., et al. "The Effect of Dietary Sodium Modification on Blood Pressure in Adults with Systolic Blood Pressure Less Than 140 mmHg: A Systematic Review." *JBI Database of Systematic Reviews and Implementation Reports* 14, no. 6 (2016): 196–237.

35. de Baaij, J. H., J. G. Hoenderop, and R. J. Bindels. "Magnesium in Man: Implications for Health and Disease." *Physiological Reviews* 95, no. 1 (2015): 1–46.

36. DiNicolantonio, J. J., J. H. O'Keefe, and W. Wilson. "Subclinical Magnesium Deficiency: A Principal Driver of Cardiovascular Disease and a Public Health Crisis." *Open Heart* 5, no. 1 (2018): e000668.

37. Guoa, W., et al. "Magnesium Deficiency on Plants: An Urgent Problem." *The Crop Journal* 4, no. 2 (2016): 83–91; Thomas, D. "The Mineral Depletion of Foods Available to Us as a Nation (1940-2002)–A Review of the 6th Edition of McCance and Widdowson." *Nutrition and Health* 19, no. 1-2 (2007): 21–55.

38. Temple, N. J. "Refined Carbohydrates—A Cause of Suboptimal Nutrient Intake." *Medical Hypotheses* 10, no. 4 (1983): 411–24.

39. Costello, R. B., et al. "Perspective: The Case for an Evidence-Based Reference Interval for Serum Magnesium: The Time Has Come." *Advances in Nutrition* 7, no. 6 (2016): 977–93.

40. Marier, J. R. "Magnesium Content of the Food Supply in the Modern-Day World." *Magnesium* 5, no. 1 (1986): 1–8.

41. Tipton, I. H., P. L. Stewart, and J. Dickson. "Patterns of Elemental Excretion in Long Term Balance Studies." *Health Physics* 16, no. 4 (1969): 455–62.

42. See note 39 above.

43. See note 36 above.

44. Rayssiguier, Y., et al. "Dietary Magnesium Affects Susceptibility of Lipoproteins and Tissues to Peroxidation in Rats." *The Journal of the American College of Nutrition* 12, no. 2 (1993): 133–7; Bussiere, L., et al. "Triglyceride-Rich Lipoproteins from Magnesium-Deficient Rats Are More Susceptible to Oxidation by Cells and Promote Proliferation of Cultured Vascular Smooth Muscle Cells." *Magnesium Research* 8, no. 2 (1995): 151–7; Turlapaty, P. D., and B. M. Altura. "Magnesium Deficiency Produces Spasms of Coronary Arteries: Relationship to Etiology of Sudden Death Ischemic Heart Disease." *Science* 208, no. 4440 (1980): 198–200.

45. See note 36 above.

46. See note 36 above.

47. Kodama, N., M. Nishimuta, and K. Suzuki. "Negative Balance of Calcium and Magnesium Under Relatively Low Sodium Intake in Humans." *Journal of Nutritional Science and Vitaminology* (Tokyo) 49, no. 3 (2003): 201–9.

48. See note 47 above.

49. Nishimuta, M., et al. "Positive Correlation Between Dietary Intake of Sodium and Balances of Calcium and Magnesium in Young Japanese Adults—Low Sodium Intake Is a Risk Factor for Loss of Calcium and Magnesium." *Journal of Nutritional Science and Vitaminology* (Tokyo) 51, no. 4 (2005): 265–70.

50. Delva, P., et al. "Intralymphocyte Free Magnesium in Patients with Primary Aldosteronism: Aldosterone and Lymphocyte Magnesium Homeostasis." *Hypertension* 35, no. 1 Pt 1 (2000): 113–7.

51. Durlach, J. "Recommended Dietary Amounts of Magnesium: Mg RDA." *Magnesium Research* 2, no. 3 (1989): 195–203.

52. See note 36 above.

53. Rosanoff, A. "Magnesium and Hypertension." *Clinical Calcium* 15, no. 2 (2005): 255–60.

54. See note 36 above.

55. Schuette, S. A., B. A. Lashner, and M. Janghorbani. "Bioavailability of Magnesium Diglycinate vs Magnesium Oxide in Patients with Ileal Resection." *Journal of Parenteral and Enteral Nutrition* 18, no. 5 (1994): 430–5.

56. Spasov, A. A., et al. "Comparative Study of Magnesium Salts Bioavailability in Rats Fed a Magnesium-Deficient Diet." *Vestnik Rossiiskoi Akademii Meditsinskikh Nauk* no. 2 (2010): 29–37; Guillard, O., et al. "Unexpected Toxicity Induced by Magnesium Orotate Treatment in Congenital Hypomagnesemia." *Journal of Internal Medicine* 252, no. 1 (2002): 88–90.

57. Ibid.

58. Phillips, R., et al. "Citrate Salts for Preventing and Treating Calcium Containing Kidney Stones in Adults." *Cochrane Database of Systematic Reviews* no. 10 (2015): Cd010057.

59. Stepura, O. B., and A. I. Martynow. "Magnesium Orotate in Severe Congestive Heart Failure (MACH)." *International Journal of Cardiology* 131, no. 2 (2009): 293–5.

Chapter 11

1. Harcombe, Z., et al. "Evidence from Randomised Controlled Trials Did Not Support the Introduction of Dietary Fat Guidelines in 1977 and 1983: A Systematic Review and Meta-Analysis." *Open Heart* 2, no. 1 (2015): e000196; Harcombe, Z., et al. "Evidence from Randomised Controlled Trials Does Not Support Current Dietary Fat Guidelines: A Systematic Review and Meta-Analysis." *Open Heart* 3, 2 (2016): e000409; DiNicolantonio, J. J. "The Cardiometabolic Consequences of Replacing Saturated Fats with Carbohydrates or Ω-6 Polyunsaturated Fats: Do the Dietary Guidelines Have It Wrong?" *Open Heart* 1 (2014): e000032. doi:10.1136/openhrt-2013-000032; Ravnskov, U., et al. "The Questionable Benefits of Exchanging Saturated Fat with Polyunsaturated Fat." *Mayo Clinic Proceedings* 89, no. 4 (2014): 451–3.

2. Teicholtz, N. *The Big Fat Surprise: Why Butter, Meat and Cheese Belong in a Healthy Diet.* New York: Simon & Schuster, 2014.

3. Barbee, M. *Politically Incorrect Nutrition: Finding Reality in the Mire of Food Industry Propaganda.* Garden City Park, NY: Square One Publishers, 2004: 27.

4. Bhupathiraju, S. N., and K. L. Tucker. "Coronary Heart Disease Prevention: Nutrients, Foods, and Dietary Patterns." *Clinica Chimica Acta* 412, no. 17–18 (2011): 1493–514.

5. Sun, Q., et al. "A Prospective Study of Trans Fatty Acids in Erythrocytes and Risk of Coronary Heart Disease." *Circulation* 115, no. 14 (2007): 1858–65; Block, R. C., et al. "Omega-6 and Trans Fatty Acids in Blood Cell Membranes: A Risk Factor for Acute Coronary Syndromes?" *American Heart Journal* 156, no. 6 (2008): 1117–23; Willett, W. C., et al. "Intake of Trans Fatty Acids and Risk of Coronary Heart Disease Among Women." *Lancet* 341, no. 8845 (1993): 581–5.

6. Grimes, W. "April 24–30; How About Some Popcorn with Your Fat?" *The New York Times*, May 1, 1994, accessed at *www.nytimes.com/1994/05/01/weekinreview/april-24-30-how-about-some-popcorn-with-your-fat.html.*

7. Hu, F. B., et al. "Dietary Fat Intake and the Risk of Coronary Heart Disease in Women." *New England Journal of Medicine* 337, no. 21 (1997): 1491–9.

8. Zaloga, G. P., et al. "Trans Fatty Acids and Coronary Heart Disease." *Nutrition in Clinical Practice* 21, no. 5 (2006): 505–12.

9. de Souza, R. J., et al. "Intake of Saturated and Trans Unsaturated Fatty Acids and Risk of All Cause Mortality, Cardiovascular Disease, and Type 2 Diabetes: Systematic Review and Meta-Analysis of Observational Studies." *The BMJ* 351 (2015): h3978.

10. See note 4 above.

11. Fox, M. "WHO Urges All Countries to Ban Trans Fats," May 14, 2018, *NBC News Health News* website, accessed at *www.nbcnews.com/health/health-news/who-urges-all-countries-ban-trans-fats-n873916.*

12. Herrera-Camacho, J., et al. "Effect of Fatty Acids on Reproductive Performance of Ruminants." June 21, 2011. Accessed at *www.intechopen.com/books/artificial-insemination-in-farm-animals/effect-of-fatty-acids-on-reproductive-performance-of-ruminants*; USDA Food Composition Databases. Accessed at *https://ndb.nal.usda.gov/ndb/.*

13. Ramsden, C. E., et al. "Use of Dietary Linoleic Acid for Secondary Prevention of Coronary Heart Disease and Death: Evaluation of Recovered Data from the Sydney Diet Heart Study and Updated Meta-Analysis." *The BMJ* 346 (2013): e8707.

14. Ramsden, C. E., et al. "n-6 Fatty Acid-Specific and Mixed Polyunsaturate Dietary Interventions Have Different Effects on CHD Risk: A Meta-Analysis of Randomised Controlled Trials." *British Journal of Nutrition* 104, no. 11 (2010): 1586–600.

15. See note 1 above.

16. Whoriskey, P. "This Study 40 Years Ago Could Have Reshaped the American Diet. But It Was Never Fully Published." *The Washington Post*, April 12, 2016, accessed at *www.washingtonpost.com/news/wonk/wp/2016/04/12/this-study-40-years-ago-could-have-reshaped-the-american-diet-but-it-was-never-fully-published/?utm_term=.2cb42d8134f2.*

17. Chowdhury, R., et al. "Association of Dietary, Circulating, and Supplement Fatty Acids with Coronary Risk: A Systematic Review and Meta-Analysis." *Annals of Internal Medicine* 160, no. 6 (2014): 398–406.

18. Siri-Tarino, P. W., et al. "Meta-Analysis of Prospective Cohort Studies Evaluating the Association of Saturated Fat with Cardiovascular Disease." *American Journal of Clinical Nutrition* 91, no. 3 (2010): 535–46.

19. Deghan, M., et al. "Associations of Fats and Carbohydrate Intake with Cardiovascular Disease and Mortality in 18 Countries from Five Continents (PURE): A Prospective Cohort Study." *The Lancet* 390, no. 10107 (2017): 2050–62.

20. Christiansen, E., et al. "Intake of a Diet High in Trans Monounsaturated Fatty Acids or Saturated Fatty Acids. Effects on Postprandial Insulinemia and Glycemia in Obese Patients with NIDDM." *Diabetes Care* 20, no. 5 (1997): 881–7.

21. Vessby, B., et al. "Substituting Dietary Saturated for Monounsaturated Fat Impairs Insulin Sensitivity in Healthy Men and Women: The KANWU Study." *Diabetologia* 44, no. 3 (2001): 312–9.

22. Piers, L. S., et al. "Substitution of Saturated with Monounsaturated Fat in a 4-Week Diet Affects Body Weight and Composition of Overweight and Obese Men." *British Journal of Nutrition* 90, no. 3 (2003): 717–27.

23. Ikemoto, S., et al. "High-Fat Diet-Induced Hyperglycemia and Obesity in Mice: Differential Effects of Dietary Oils." *Metabolism* 45, no. 12 (1996): 1539–46.

24. Kien, C. L., J. Y. Bunn, and F. Ugrasbul. "Increasing Dietary Palmitic Acid Decreases Fat Oxidation and Daily Energy Expenditure." *American Journal of Clinical Nutrition* 82, no. 2 (2005): 320–6.

25. Kastorini, C. M., et al. "The Effect of Mediterranean Diet on Metabolic Syndrome and Its Components: A Meta-Analysis of 50 Studies and 534,906 Individuals." *Journal of the American College of Cardiology* 57, no. 11 (2011): 1299–313.

26. Jones, P. J., P. B. Pencharz, and M. T. Clandinin. "Whole Body Oxidation of Dietary Fatty Acids: Implications for Energy Utilization." *American Journal of Clinical Nutrition* 42, no. 5 (1985): 769–77.

27. Piers, L. S., et al. "The Influence of the Type of Dietary Fat on Postprandial Fat Oxidation Rates: Monounsaturated (Olive Oil) Vs Saturated Fat (Cream)." *International Journal of Obesity and Related Metabolic Disorders* 26, no. 6 (2002): 814–21.

28. Kien, C. L., and J. Y. Bunn. "Gender Alters the Effects of Palmitate and Oleate on Fat Oxidation and Energy Expenditure." *Obesity* (Silver Spring) 16, no. 1 (2008): 29–33.

29. Soares, M. J., et al. "The Acute Effects of Olive Oil V. Cream on Postprandial Thermogenesis and Substrate Oxidation in Postmenopausal Women." *British Journal of Nutrition* 91, no. 2 (2004): 245–52.

30. Piers, L. S., et al. "Substitution of Saturated with Monounsaturated Fat in a 4-Week Diet Affects Body Weight and Composition of Overweight and Obese Men." *British Journal of Nutrition* 90, no. 3 (2003): 717–27; Piers, L. S., et al. "The Influence of the Type of Dietary Fat on Postprandial Fat Oxidation Rates: Monounsaturated (Olive Oil) Vs Saturated Fat (Cream)." *International Journal of Obesity and Related Metabolic Disorders* 26, no. 6 (2002): 814–21; Thomsen, C., et al. "Differential Effects of Saturated and Monounsaturated Fats on Postprandial Lipemia and Glucagon-Like Peptide 1 Responses in Patients with Type 2 Diabetes." *American Journal of Clinical Nutrition* 77, no. 3 (2003): 605–11; Thomsen, C., et al. "Differential Effects of Saturated and Monounsaturated Fatty Acids on Postprandial Lipemia and Incretin Responses in Healthy Subjects." *American Journal of Clinical Nutrition* 69, no. 6 (1999): 1135–43.

31. Feranil, A. B., et al. "Coconut Oil Is Associated with a Beneficial Lipid Profile in Pre-Menopausal Women in the Philippines." *Asia Pacific Journal of Clinical Nutrition* 20, no. 2 (2011): 190–5.

32. Babu, A. S., et al. "Virgin Coconut Oil and Its Potential Cardioprotective Effects." *Postgrad Medicine* 126, no. 7 (2014): 76–83.

33. St-Onge, M. P., et al. "Medium Chain Triglyceride Oil Consumption as Part of a Weight Loss Diet Does Not Lead to an Adverse Metabolic Profile When Compared to Olive Oil." *The Journal of the American College of Nutrition* 27, no. 5 (2008): 547–52.

34. Nosaka, N., et al. "Effects of Margarine Containing Medium-Chain Triacylglycerols on Body Fat Reduction in Humans." *Journal of Atherosclerosis and Thrombosis* 10, no. 5 (2003): 290–8.

35. Stubbs, R. J., and C. G. Harbron. "Covert Manipulation of the Ratio of Medium- to Long-Chain Triglycerides in Isoenergetically Dense Diets: Effect on Food Intake in Ad Libitum Feeding Men." *International Journal of Obesity and Related Metabolic Disorders* 20, no. 5 (1996): 435–44.

36. Van Wymelbeke, V., et al. "Influence of Medium-Chain and Long-Chain Triacylglycerols on the Control of Food Intake in Men." *American Journal of Clinical Nutrition* 68, no. 2 (1998): 226–34.

37. Scalfi, L., A. Coltorti, and F. Contaldo. "Postprandial Thermogenesis in Lean and Obese Subjects After Meals Supplemented with Medium-Chain and Long-Chain Triglycerides." *American Journal of Clinical Nutrition* 53, no. 5 (1991): 1130–3.

38. Heid, M. "You Asked: Is Coconut Oil Healthy?" *Time*, April 26, 2017, accessed at *www.time.com/4755761/coconut-oil-healthy/*.

39. St-Onge, M. P., and P. J. Jones. "Physiological Effects of Medium-Chain Triglycerides: Potential Agents in the Prevention of Obesity." *The Journal of Nutrition* 132, no. 3 (2002): 329–32.

40. Lindeberg, S., and B. Lundh. "Apparent Absence of Stroke and Ischaemic Heart Disease in a Traditional Melanesian Island: A Clinical Study in Kitava." *Journal of Internal Medicine* 233, no. 3 (1993): 269–75.

41. Stanhope, J. M., and I. A. Prior. "The Tokelau Island Migrant Study: Prevalence and Incidence of Diabetes Mellitus." *New Zealand Medical Journal* 92, no. 673 (1980): 417–21.

42. de Oliveira Otto, M. C., et al. "Serial Measures of Circulating Biomarkers of Dairy Fat and Total and Cause-Specific Mortality in Older Adults: The Cardiovascular Health Study." *American Journal of Clinical Nutrition* 108, no. 3 (2018): 476–84.

43. Yakoob, M. Y., et al. "Circulating Biomarkers of Dairy Fat and Risk of Incident Stroke in U.S. Men and Women in 2 Large Prospective Cohorts." *American Journal of Clinical Nutrition* 100, no. 6 (2014): 1437–47.

44. University of Texas Health Science Center at Houston. "New Research Could Banish Guilty Feeling for Consuming Whole Dairy Products." *Science Daily* website, accessed at *www.sciencedaily.com/releases/2018/07/180711182735.htm*.

45. Aune, D., et al. "Dairy Products and the Risk of Type 2 Diabetes: A Systematic Review and Dose-Response Meta-Analysis of Cohort Studies." *American Journal of Clinical Nutrition* 98, no. 4 (2013): 1066–83.

46. Astrup, A. "A Changing View on Saturated Fatty Acids and Dairy: From Enemy to Friend." *American Journal of Clinical Nutrition* 100, no. 6 (2014): 1407–8.

47. Freeman, A. M., et al. "Trending Cardiovascular Nutrition Controversies." *Journal of the American College of Cardiology* 69, no. 9 (2017): 1172–87.

48. Eckel, R. H., et al. "2013 AHA/ACC Guideline on Lifestyle Management to Reduce Cardiovascular Risk: A Report of the American College of Cardiology/American Heart Association Task Force on Practice Guidelines. *Journal of the American College of Cardiology* 63, no. 25 Pt B (2014): 2960–84.

49. Covas, M. I., et al. "The Effect of Polyphenols in Olive Oil on Heart Disease Risk Factors: A Randomized Trial." *Annals of Internal Medicine* 145, no. 5 (2006): 333–41.

50. Wiseman, S. A., et al. "Dietary Non-Tocopherol Antioxidants Present in Extra Virgin Olive Oil Increase the Resistance of Low Density Lipoproteins to Oxidation in Rabbits." *Atherosclerosis* 120, no. 1–2 (1996): 15–23; Caruso, D., et al. "Effect of Virgin Olive Oil Phenolic Compounds on In Vitro Oxidation of Human Low Density Lipoproteins." *Nutrition, Metabolism and Cardiovascular Diseases* 9, no. 3 (1999): 102–7; Coni, E., et al. "Protective Effect of Oleuropein, an Olive Oil Biophenol, on Low Density Lipoprotein Oxidizability in Rabbits." *Lipids* 35, no. 1 (2000): 45–54.

51. Aviram, M., and K. Eias. "Dietary Olive Oil Reduces Low-Density Lipoprotein Uptake by Macrophages and Decreases the Susceptibility of the Lipoprotein to Undergo Lipid Peroxidation." *Annals of Nutrition and Metabolism* 37, no. 2 (1993): 75–84.

52. Bogani, P., et al. "Postprandial Anti-Inflammatory and Antioxidant Effects of Extra Virgin Olive Oil." *Atherosclerosis* 190, no. 1 (2007): 181–6.

53. Pacheco, Y. M., et al. "Minor Compounds of Olive Oil Have Postprandial Anti-Inflammatory Effects." *British Journal of Nutrition* 98, no. 2 (2007): 260–3.

54. Fabiani, R., et al. "Oxidative DNA Damage Is Prevented by Extracts of Olive Oil, Hydroxytyrosol, and Other Olive Phenolic Compounds in Human Blood Mononuclear Cells and HL60 Cells." *The Journal of Nutrition* 138, no. 8 (2008): 1411–6.

55. Moreno-Luna, R., et al. "Olive Oil Polyphenols Decrease Blood Pressure and Improve Endothelial Function in Young Women with Mild Hypertension." *American Journal of Hypertension* 25, no. 12 (2012): 1299–304.

56. DiNicolantonio, J. J., et al. "Omega-3s and Cardiovascular Health." *Ochsner Journal* 14, no. 3 (2014): 399–412.

57. DiNicolantonio, J. J., P. Meier, and J. H. O'Keefe. "Omega-3 Polyunsaturated Fatty Acids for the Prevention of Cardiovascular Disease: Do Formulation, Dosage & Comparator Matter?" *Missouri Medicine* 110, no. 6 (2013): 495–8.

58. Hulbert, A. J., and P. L. Else. "Membranes as Possible Pacemakers of Metabolism." *Journal of Theoretical Biology* 199, no. 3 (1999): 257–74; Smith, G. I., et al. "Dietary Omega-3 Fatty Acid Supplementation Increases the Rate of Muscle Protein Synthesis in Older Adults: A Randomized Controlled Trial." *American Journal of Clinical Nutrition* 93, no. 2 (2011): 402–12; Whitehouse, A. S., et al. "Mechanism of Attenuation of Skeletal Muscle Protein Catabolism in Cancer Cachexia by Eicosapentaenoic Acid." *Cancer Research* 61, no. 9 (2001): 3604–9.

59. See note 29 above.

60. Deutsch, L. "Evaluation of the Effect of Neptune Krill Oil on Chronic Inflammation and Arthritic Symptoms." *The Journal of the American College of Nutrition* 26, no. 1 (2007): 39–48.

61. Sampalis, F., et al. "Evaluation of the Effects of Neptune Krill Oil in the Management of Premenstrual Syndrome and Dysmenorrhea." *Alternative Medicine Review* 8, no. 2 (2003): 171–9.

62. Bunea, R., K. El Farrah, and L. Deutsch. "Evaluation of the Effects of Neptune Krill Oil on the Clinical Course of Hyperlipidemia." *Alternative Medicine Review* 9, no. 4 (2004): 420–8.

63. Bower, B. "Human Ancestors Had Taste for Meat, Brains." *Science News*, May 3, 2013, accessed at *www.sciencenews.org/article/human-ancestors-had-taste-meat-brains*.

64. Cordain, L., et al. "Fatty Acid Analysis of Wild Ruminant Tissues: Evolutionary Implications for Reducing Diet-Related Chronic Disease." *European Journal of Clinical Nutrition* 56, no. 3 (2002): 181–91.

65. Nguyen, L. N., et al. "Mfsd2a Is a Transporter for the Essential Omega-3 Fatty Acid Docosahexaenoic Acid." *Nature* 509, no. 7501 (2014): 503–6; Alakbarzade, V., et al. "A Partially Inactivating Mutation in the Sodium-Dependent Lysophosphatidylcholine Transporter MFSD2A Causes a Non-Lethal Microcephaly Syndrome." *Nature Genetics* 47, no. 7 (2015): 814–7; Guemez-Gamboa, A., et al. "Inactivating Mutations in MFSD2A, Required for Omega-3 Fatty Acid Transport in Brain, Cause a Lethal Microcephaly Syndrome." *Nature Genetics* 47, no. 7 (2015): 809–13.

66. Bunea, R., K. El Farrah, and L. Deutsch. "Evaluation of the Effects of Neptune Krill Oil on the Clinical Course of Hyperlipidemia." *Alternative Medicine Review* 9, no. 4 (2004): 420–8; "Neptune Krill Oil." Accessed at *https://nutrisan-export.com/wp-content/uploads/2016/03/productinfoNKO.pdf*; Batetta, B., et al. "Endocannabinoids May Mediate the Ability of (n-3) Fatty Acids to Reduce Ectopic Fat and Inflammatory Mediators in Obese Zucker Rats." *The Journal of Nutrition* 139, 8 (2009): 1495–501; Nishida, Y., et al. "Quenching Activities of Common Hydrophilic and Lipophilic Antioxidants Against Singlet Oxygen Using Chemiluminescence Detection System." *Carotenoid Science* 11, no. 6 (2007): 16–20; "This Powerhouse Antioxidant Slips Through Your Cell Membranes with Ease to Help Protect Your Brain, Heart, Eyes, Lungs, Muscles, Joints, Skin, Mitochondria and More... Are You Getting Enough?" *Dr. Mercola* website, accessed at *https://products.mercola.com/astaxanthin/*

Chapter 12

1. Miyagi, S., et al. "Longevity and Diet in Okinawa, Japan: The Past, Present and Future." *Asia Pacific Journal of Public Health* 15 Suppl (2003): S3–9.

2. Willcox, D. C., et al. "The Okinawan Diet: Health Implications of a Low-Calorie, Nutrient-Dense, Antioxidant-Rich Dietary Pattern Low in Glycemic Load." *The Journal of the American College of Nutrition* 28 Suppl (2009): 500s–516s.

3. Sho, H. "History and Characteristics of Okinawan Longevity Food." *Asia Pacific Journal of Clinical Nutrition* 10, no. 2 (2001): 159–64.

4. Willcox, B. J., et al. "Caloric Restriction, the Traditional Okinawan Diet, and Healthy Aging: The Diet of The World's Longest-Lived People and Its Potential Impact on Morbidity and Life Span." *Annals of the New York Academy of Sciences* 1114 (2007): 434–55.

5. See note 2 above.

6. See note 4 above.

7. "The Elixir of Life." *The Daily Dish* website, accessed at *www.theatlantic.com/daily-dish/archive/2007/10/the-elixir-of-life/224942/*.

8. Poulain, M., et al. "Identification of a Geographic Area Characterized by Extreme Longevity in the Sardinia Island: The AKEA Study." *Experimental Gerontology* 39, no. 9 (2004): 1423–9.

9. Pes, G. M., et al. "Male Longevity in Sardinia, a Review of Historical Sources Supporting a Causal Link with Dietary Factors." *European Journal of Clinical Nutrition* 69, no. 4 (2015): 411–8.

10. Rizzo, N. S., et al. "Vegetarian Dietary Patterns Are Associated with a Lower Risk of Metabolic Syndrome: The Adventist Health Study 2." *Diabetes Care* 34, no. 5 (2011): 1225–7; Tantamango-Bartley, Y., et al. "Vegetarian Diets and the Incidence of Cancer in a Low-Risk Population." *Cancer Epidemiology, Biomarkers & Prevention* 22, no. 2 (2013): 286–94.

11. Kiani, F., et al. "Dietary Risk Factors for Ovarian Cancer: The Adventist Health Study (United States)." *Cancer Causes & Control* 17, no. 2 (2006): 137–46; "The Adventist Health Study: Findings for Cancer." Loma Linda University School of Public Health, accessed at *https://publichealth.llu.edu/adventist-health-studies/findings/findings-past-studies/adventist-health-study-findings-cancer*.

12. Buettner, D. *The Blue Zones Solution: Eating and Living Like the World's Healthiest People*. Washington, D.C.: National Geographic Society (2015).

13. Rosero-Bixby, L., W. H. Dow, and D. H. Rehkopf. "The Nicoya Region of Costa Rica: A High Longevity Island for Elderly Males." *Vienna Yearbook of Population Research* 11 (2013): 109–36.

14. Shah, Y. "5 Things the Greeks Can Teach Us About Aging Well." *The Huffington Post*, December 6, 2017, accessed at *www.huffingtonpost.com/2014/04/22/longevity-greece-_n_5128337.html*.

15. Buettner, D. "The Island Where People Forget to Die." *The New York Times*, October 28, 2012, accessed at *www.nytimes.com/2012/10/28/magazine/the-island-where-people-forget-to-die.html*.

16. Ibid.

17. Sarri, K. O., et al. "Effects of Greek Orthodox Christian Church Fasting on Serum Lipids and Obesity." *BMC Public Health* 3 (2003): 16.

18. Shikany, J. M., et al. "Southern Dietary Pattern Is Associated with Hazard of Acute Coronary Heart Disease in the Reasons for Geographic and Racial Differences in Stroke (REGARDS) Study." *Circulation* 132, no. 9 (2015): 804–14.

19. Alles, B., et al. "Comparison of Sociodemographic and Nutritional Characteristics Between Self-Reported Vegetarians, Vegans, and Meat-Eaters from the NutriNet-Sante Study." *Nutrients* 9, no. 9 (2017): E1023.

20. Martins, M. C. T., et al. "A New Approach to Assess Lifetime Dietary Patterns Finds Lower Consumption of Animal Foods with Aging in a Longitudinal Analysis of a Health-Oriented Adventist Population." *Nutrients* 9, no. 10 (2017): E1118.

21. Davis, C., et al. "Definition of the Mediterranean Diet; a Literature Review." *Nutrients* 7, no. 11 (2015): 9139–53.

INDEX

M

macronutrients, 46

magnesium
about, 147, 160–161, 163
deficiency in, 162
salt and, 161–162
as step 4 in plan for healthy aging, 215–216
supplemental, 162–163

mammalian target of rapamycin (mTOR), 40–41

marasmus, 53

marine omega-3 fats, 185, 186–187

McCay, Clive, 25

MCTs (medium-chain triglycerides), 180–182

meat
about, 70–71
in Okinawa, Japan, 193
in Sardinia, Italy, 196–197

MEDIS study, 124–125

Mediterranean diet, 179

medium-chain triglycerides (MCTs), 180–182

Meneely, G. R., 149

metabolic sink, 86

metazoans, 15

methionine, 57

Minnesota Coronary Experiment, 176

Mithridates VI, 19–21

Mitochondrial Theory, 19

monounsaturated fats, 170–171, 178–179, 180

monounsaturated fatty acids (MUFAs), 178–179

Mozaffarian, Dariush, 177

mTOR
about, 33–34, 40–41, 46–48
reducing, 48
as step 2 in plan for healthy aging, 211–213

MUFAs (monounsaturated fatty acids), 178–179

muscle atrophy, 19

muscle protein synthesis, 88–89

N

N-acetylcysteine (NAC), 68

National Health and Nutrition Examination Survey (NHANES), 154

Nicoya Peninsula, Costa Rica, 200

nitric oxide (NO), 140

Nógrády, Georges, 39

nonresistance training, 213

Normative Aging Study, 140

nutrient sensors, 30–32

Nutrition Facts Label, 149

nuts, 75, 183–184

O

obesity, 50, 122–125

Okinawa, Japan, 27, 192–195

Okinawan people, 27

oleic acid, 179, 183

olive oil, 184–185

omega-3 fatty acids, 87, 171, 173–174, 185, 186–187

omega-6 fats, 170, 173–174

oolong tea, 123

Organic Traditions, 67, 163, 181, 184, 185

Orlistat, 122

osteoblasts, 55

osteoclasts, 55

osteoporosis, 14, 80

oxidation rate, 179

oxidized linoleic acid metabolites (OXLAMs), 175

P

Pacific salmon, 17

Parkinson's disease, 14

partially hydrogenated oils, 169

Peterson, Jordan, 63

phytochemicals, 73

PI3K pathway, 31